Get ahead!

surgery

100 EMQs for Finals

Second edition

Get ahead!

surgery

100 EMQs for Finals

Second edition

James Wigley MBBS BSc MRCS AFHEA
University Hospital Southampton, Southampton, UK

Saran Shantikumar MRCS, BHF Clinical Fellow
Bristol Heart Institute, Bristol, UK

CRC Press
Taylor & Francis Group
Boca Raton London New York

CRC Press is an imprint of the
Taylor & Francis Group, an **informa** business

CRC Press
Taylor & Francis Group
6000 Broken Sound Parkway NW, Suite 300
Boca Raton, FL 33487-2742

First issued in hardback 2017

Version Date: 20140826

ISBN-13: 978-1-4441-8180-7 (pbk)
ISBN-13: 978-1-138-45139-1 (hbk)

Visit the Taylor & Francis Web site at
http://www.taylorandfrancis.com

and the CRC Press Web site at
http://www.crcpress.com

Contents

Preface

Welcome to *Get ahead! SURGERY.* This book contains 100 EMQ themes, each with five stems, arranged as six practice papers lasting two hours apiece. You can either work through the practice papers systematically or dip in and out of the book using the EMQ theme titles as a guide to where questions on a specific topic can be found. We have tried to include all the surgical conditions about which you can be expected to know, as well as some more detailed knowledge suitable for candidates aiming towards distinction. As in the real exam, these papers have no preset pass mark. Whether you pass or fail depends on the distribution of scores across the whole year group, but around 60% should be sufficient.

We hope this book fulfils its aim in being a useful, informative revision aid. If you have any feedback or suggestions, please let us know (RevisionForMedicalFinals@gmail.com).

We would also like to acknowledge the help of Stephen Clausard, Development Editor at CRC Press, for his patience and proactivity in commissioning and supporting this edition and others in the *Get ahead!* series.

James Wigley
Saran Shantikumar

Introduction to *Get ahead!*

GET AHEAD!

Extended matching questions (EMQs) are becoming more popular as a method of assessment in summative medical school examinations. EMQs have the advantage of testing candidates' knowledge of clinical scenarios rather than their ability at detailed factual recall. However, they do not always parallel real-life situations and are no comparison to clinical decision making. Either way, the EMQ is here to stay.

The *Get ahead!* series is aimed primarily at undergraduate finalists. Much like the real exam, we have endeavoured to include commonly asked questions as well as a generous proportion of harder stems, appropriate for the more ambitious student aiming for honours. The Medical Schools Council Assessment Alliance (MSCAA) is a partnership aiming to improve assessment practice between all undergraduate medical schools in the UK. The questions in the *Get ahead!* series are written to follow the style of the MSCAA EMQs, and hence are of a similar format to what many of you can expect in your exams. All the questions in the *Get ahead!* series are accompanied by explanatory answers, including a succinct summary of the key features of each condition. Even when you get an answer right, I strongly suggest you read these – I guarantee you'll learn something. For added interest, we have included details of eponymous persons ('eponymous' from Greek *epi* = upon + *onyma* = name; 'giving name'), and, as you have just seen, some derivations of words from the original Latin or Greek.

HOW TO PASS YOUR EXAMS

Exam EMQs are intended to be based on 'house officer knowledge'. Sadly, this is not always the case, and you shouldn't be surprised when you get a question concerning the management of various stages of prostate cancer (as I was). So start revising early and don't restrict yourself to the given syllabus if you can avoid it. If your exam is only two weeks away then CRAM, CRAM, CRAM – you'll be surprised at how much you can learn in a fortnight.

During the exam...

1. Try to answer the questions without looking at the responses first – the questions are written such that this should be possible.

2. Take your time to read the questions fully. There are no bonus marks for finishing the paper early.
3. If you get stuck on a question then make sure you mark down your best guess before you move on. You may not have time to return to it at the end.
4. Answer all the questions – there is no negative marking. If you are unsure, go with your instinct – it's probably going to be your best guess.
5. Never think that the examiner is trying to catch you out. Red herrings are not allowed, so don't assume there is one. If a question looks easy, it probably is!

But all this is obvious and there is no substitute for learning the material thoroughly and practising as many questions as you can. With this book, you're off to a good start!

A final word...

The *Get ahead!* series is written by junior doctors who have recently finished finals and who have experience teaching students. As such, I hope the books cover information that is valuable and relevant to you as undergraduates who are about to sit finals.

I wish you the best of luck in your exams!

Saran Shantikumar
Series Editor, Get ahead!

Practice Paper 1: Questions

THEME 1: INVESTIGATION OF ABDOMINAL PAIN

Options

A. CT scan
B. Erect chest X-ray
C. Faecal elastase level
D. Laparoscopy
E. Mesenteric angiography
F. Serum amylase
G. Supine chest X-ray
H. Troponin levels
I. Urgent laparotomy

For each of the following people presenting with abdominal pain, select the next appropriate investigation. Each option may be used once, more than once or not at all.

1. A 29-year-old man is admitted to the emergency department with sudden-onset, severe abdominal pain radiating to the back and with vomiting. On examination, there is tenderness and guarding in the epigastrium. His pulse is 118 beats/min and his blood pressure is 96/68 mmHg.
2. A 74-year-old woman with a history of osteoarthritis presents with acute severe abdominal pain and vomiting. On examination, the abdomen is rigid and bowel sounds are absent.
3. A 24-year-old woman presents with sudden-onset right iliac fossa pain with nausea and vomiting. She was admitted last year with similar symptoms, which turned out to be torsion of an ovarian cyst. Examination reveals tenderness and guarding in the right iliac fossa.
4. A 69-year-old man presents with a 2-month history of severe central abdominal pain occurring 20 minutes after eating. He is reluctant to eat nowadays and has dropped a waist size. He has a medical history of intermittent claudication. Examination of the abdomen is unremarkable.
5. A 69-year-old man with a long history of gastro-oesophageal reflux presents with worsening dysphagia to solids, epigastric discomfort and weight loss. An urgent endoscopy shows a mass lesion in the lower third of the oesophagus.

THEME 2: BURNS

Options

A. 1%
B. 9%
C. 10%
D. 18%
E. 19%
F. 27%
G. 36%
H. 37%
I. 45%
J. 54%

For each of the following scenarios, estimate the percentage burn area. Each option may be used once, more than once or not at all.

1. A 54-year-old man with burns to his right upper limb.
2. A 72-year-old man with burns to his left lower limb and left upper limb.
3. A 34-year-old woman with burns to her head and neck and anterior torso.
4. A 62-year-old man with burns to his right lower limb and perineum.
5. A 37-year-old woman with burns to her head and neck, right upper limb, left palm, and posterior torso.

THEME 3: BACK PAIN

Options

A. Central intervertebral disc herniation
B. Coccydynia
C. Discitis
D. Posterolateral intervertebral disc herniation
E. Pott's disease
F. Spinal stenosis
G. Spondylolisthesis
H. Spondylolysis
I. Spondylosis

For each of the following presentations, select the most likely diagnosis. Each option may be used once, more than once or not at all.

1. A 37-year-old builder presents with sudden-onset back pain that radiates down his leg to his foot. On examination, he has a reduced straight leg raise. Neurological examination is unremarkable.
2. A 52-year-old lorry driver presents with a 2-year history of backache, which originally started when he fell out of his truck. The pain is present every day and is worse after standing for long periods. On examination,

there is mild tenderness over the lower back. Straight leg raise and neurological examination show no abnormality.

3. A 62-year-old man presents with a 4-month history of back pain and calf pain that occurs on walking. The pain eventually resolves when activity is ceased. It is also relieved by leaning forwards. Peripheral vascular and neurological examinations are within normal limits.
4. A 4-year-old girl is brought in by her mother, as she has been refusing to walk all day. She is extremely irritable, and percussion over her lower spine causes her to start crying. Lower limb examination is unremarkable.
5. A 32-year-old man presents with a 6-month history of lower back pain that occasionally radiates down his leg. The pain is worse when standing. On examination, a 'step' is palpable above the sacral crest.

THEME 4: INTESTINAL OBSTRUCTION

Options

A. Adhesions
B. Bezoar
C. Colonic malignancy
D. Crohn's disease stricture
E. Faecal impaction
F. Gallstone ileus
G. Intussusception
H. Paralytic ileus
I. Sigmoid volvulus
J. Strangulated hernia

For each of the following people presenting with intestinal obstruction, select the most likely diagnosis. Each option may be used once, more than once or not at all.

1. A 72-year-old man presents with abdominal pain and distension. On examination, the pain is worse in the lower abdomen. An abdominal X-ray shows a single loop of dilated bowel that turns back on itself.
2. A 42-year-old woman presents with a 24-hour history of central abdominal pain and vomiting. On examination, she has a midline laparotomy scar but no other abnormality.
3. A 72-year-old woman presents with a 12-hour history of colicky abdominal pain and distension. An abdominal X-ray shows multiple loops of dilated small bowel and gas in the biliary tree.
4. A 66-year-old man underwent a semi-elective bowel resection for a caecal tumour 2 days ago. You are called to see him as he is vomiting and has not passed flatus since the operation. On examination, his abdomen is distended but non-tender. Bowel sounds are absent.

5. A 14-year-old girl is brought by her parents to the emergency department with a 12-month history of indigestion, nausea and stomach upsets. She has a history of psychiatric problems, for which she is under regular follow-up. Abdominal examination is unremarkable. A barium swallow shows an irregular, round filling defect in the duodenum.

THEME 5: ULCERS

Options

A. Arterial ulcer
B. Cushing ulcer
C. Marjolin ulcer
D. Martorell ulcer
E. Necrobiosis lipoidica
F. Neuropathic ulcer
G. Rodent ulcer
H. Syphilitic ulcer
I. Venous ulcer

For each of the following presentations, select the most likely diagnosis. Each option may be used once, more than once or not at all.

1. A 72-year-old man attends his general practice with a cramping pain in his buttocks that occurs on walking. When he develops the cramps, he has to rest until they disappear. On examination, it is difficult to feel his distal lower limb pulses. On the dorsal left foot is a deep, sharply defined ulcer that the patient finds painful.
2. A 62-year-old woman presents to her general practitioner with a raised, pink papule on her left arm. On examination, you note that the lesion is painless and firm, and arises from an underlying scar. She mentions that the scar was from a burn injury that happened 20 years ago.
3. A 62-year-old man presents with a painless lesion on his right cheek that has been present for over a month. On examination, the lesion is raised and flesh-coloured with central ulceration. There is no evidence of pigmentation.
4. A 34-year-old woman attends her regular diabetes clinic with an ulcer on the sole of her right foot. On examination, the foot is warm and peripheral pulses are palpable. The ulcer itself is deep and painless and you find that she has sensory loss below the ankles bilaterally.
5. An 18-year-old man presents to the emergency department with multiple painless ulcers over his arms and legs. He also complains of a fever, malaise and a sore throat. On examination, you note widespread lymphadenopathy. The patient tells you that he originally had a single painless ulcer in his groin but this resolved spontaneously.

THEME 6: MANAGEMENT OF HERNIAS

Options

A. Elective repair
B. Emergency repair
C. Observation only
D. Prompt repair
E. Urgent repair

For each of the following presentations, select the most appropriate management. Each option may be used once, more than once or not at all.

1. A 54-year-old man has a long-standing hernia above and medial to the pubic tubercle that does not descend into the scrotum. The hernia is easily reducible and the patient is asymptomatic.
2. A 75-year-old woman has a hernia in her left groin that is below and lateral to the pubic tubercle. On examination, the hernia is tender, erythematous and irreducible, and the patient is complaining of colicky abdominal pain and vomiting.
3. A 47-year-old man has a hernia that is above and medial to the pubic tubercle and descends into the scrotum on standing. On examination, the hernia is reducible and the patient is asymptomatic.
4. A 62-year-old woman has a hernia that is below and lateral to the pubic tubercle. On examination, the patient is well and the hernia is painless but irreducible.
5. A 57-year-old man has a scrotal hernia that has only been present for a fortnight. On examination, the hernia is irreducible but painless.

THEME 7: DIAGNOSIS OF BREAST DISEASE

Options

A. Breast cancer
B. Breast cyst
C. Duct ectasia
D. Fat necrosis
E. Fibroroadenoma
F. Fibrocystic disease
G. Galactocele
H. Gynaecomastia
I. Lactating breast
J. Paget disease
K. Peau d'orange
L. Phyllodes tumour
M. Prolactinoma

For each of the following people presenting with breast disease, select the most likely diagnosis. Each option may be used once, more than once or not at all.

1. A 17-year-old female presents with multiple bilateral cystic swellings, which she admits to having for years. These are causing her considerable discomfort, especially premenstrually.
2. A woman of 25 years presents to her general practitioner with a single 4 cm firm, smooth lump in the upper outer quadrant of the breast. On examination, it is noted that the lump is not adherent to the overlying skin and is freely mobile within the breast.
3. A 42-year-old woman attends the breast clinic with a rapidly growing irregular mass in her right breast. On examination, it is 6 cm in diameter. Core biopsy later reveals mixed epithelial and connective tissue elements.
4. A 62-year-old woman complains of dry, cracked skin around the right areola. On examination, there is a discrete firm nodule underlying the affected area.
5. A 72-year-old woman went to her general practitioner complaining of a swelling in the left breast. On examination, you notice dimpling of the skin in the left breast and a firm 3 cm lump in the lower outer quadrant.

THEME 8: MANAGEMENT OF TESTICULAR CONDITIONS

Options

A. Antibiotics
B. Aspiration of fluid
C. Chemotherapy alone
D. Excision of cyst
E. Herniorrhaphy
F. Orchidectomy alone
G. Orchidectomy + chemotherapy
H. Orchidectomy + radiotherapy
I. Orchidectomy + radiotherapy + chemotherapy
J. Radiotherapy alone
K. Reassurance and simple analgesia
L. Reduction and fixation

For each of the following scenarios, select the most appropriate management. Each option may be used once, more than once or not at all.

1. An 18-year-old man presents with a swelling in his left testicle. On examination, the swelling is tense, smooth, fluctuant and transilluminates. The testis cannot be felt separate to the swelling. The patient wants treatment for this swelling.
2. A 10-year-old boy presents with sudden-onset pain and swelling in his left testicle. On examination, the left testicle lies higher than the right, is erythematous and is exquisitely tender.

3. A 42-year-old man presents with a painless lump in his right scrotum that he first noticed last week. On examination, the swelling is hard and irregular and does not transilluminate. A CT scan rules out lymph node involvement.
4. A 37-year-old man presents with a 2-day history of pain and swelling in his right testicle and pain on passing water. On examination, his left scrotum is swollen, erythematous and tender. Urine dipstick shows white cells.
5. A 23-year-old man presents with pain and swelling in his scrotum. On examination, a hard, irregular mass is felt in the left scrotum that does not transilluminate. A CT scan demonstrates the presence of enlarged para-aortic lymph nodes.

THEME 9: HYPERSENSITIVITY REACTIONS

Options

A. Type I hypersensitivity
B. Type II hypersensitivity
C. Type III hypersensitivity
D. Type IV hypersensitivity
E. Type V hypersensitivity

For each of the following presentations, select the most appropriate type of hypersensitivity reaction. Each option may be used once, more than once or not at all.

1. A 12-year-old boy develops sudden-onset wheezing, tongue swelling and a widespread rash following ingestion of a peanut butter sandwich.
2. A 22-year-old woman presents with a short history of haematuria. A urine dipstick confirmed the presence of microscopic haematuria and proteinuria. The patient admits to having some time off university earlier in the month with a sore throat.
3. A 34-year-old woman presents with a 4-week history of diarrhoea, weight loss and feeling warm. On examination, she has a diffuse midline neck swelling.
4. A 47-year-old woman presents with itching and redness on both ear lobes where she has started wearing new earrings.
5. A 32-year-old multiparous woman gives birth to a stillborn baby. The mother was known to be Rhesus-negative and the baby was found to be Rhesus-positive.

THEME 10: NECK LUMPS

Options

A. Acute bacterial sialolithiasis
B. Branchial cyst
C. Chemodectoma

D. Cystic hygroma
E. Pleomorphic adenoma
F. Salivary duct carcinoma
G. Salivary gland stone
H. Sternocleidomastoid tumour
I. Thyroglossal cyst
J. Virchow's node

For each of the following people with neck lumps, select the most likely diagnosis. Each option may be used once, more than once or not at all.

1. A 1-year-old boy is brought to the general practice by his mother with a large mass in his neck that has been present for a while. On examination, the mass is posterior to the left sternocleidomastoid muscle. It is fleshy, compressible and transilluminates.
2. A 64-year-old woman presents with a rapidly growing mass in her neck associated with a drooping of the right side of her face. On examination, there is a 4 cm hard mass in the neck that is attached to the overlying skin.
3. A 13-year-old boy presents with a painless neck lump on the left side. On examination, there is a 2 cm lump at the anterior border of sternocleidomastoid that is smooth and fluctuant but does not transilluminate.
4. An 8-year-old girl presents with a smooth lump in the midline of the neck. On examination, there is a 1 cm painless, fluctuant swelling in the midline that moves up on swallowing and with tongue protrusion.
5. A 56-year-old man presents to the emergency department with a pain and swelling in his neck that occurs every time he eats and lasts around an hour. He has experienced this for over a fortnight. On examination, there is no obvious swelling or erythema.

THEME 11: CLASSIFICATION OF JAUNDICE

Options

A. Pre-hepatic
B. Hepatic
C. Post-hepatic

For each of the following scenarios choose the term that best describes the origin of jaundice. Each option may be used once, more than once or not at all.

1. A 25-year-old mature student decides to enter a drug trial to fund his education. Routine blood tests on admission show an elevated bilirubin concentration in the absence of any other abnormality.
2. A 39-year-old man develops jaundice after commencing rifampicin and isoniazid for tuberculosis.
3. A 65-year-old woman is started on a blood transfusion after a lower gastrointestinal bleed secondary to angiodysplasia. A short while into the transfusion, she develops fever, shortness of breath and jaundice.

4. A 48-year-old woman presents with right upper quadrant pain, nausea and jaundice. On further questioning, she admits to having pale stools and dark urine.
5. A 36-year-old man returns from travelling around Southeast Asia and develops diarrhoea and vomiting. A couple of days later, he suffers abdominal pains and notices that his eyes are becoming yellow.

THEME 12: SHOULDER DISORDERS

Options

A. Anterior dislocation
B. Frozen shoulder
C. Impingement syndrome
D. Posterior dislocation
E. Rotator cuff tear
F. Rupture of long head of biceps
G. Supraspinatus tendonitis

For each of the following people presenting with shoulder problems, select the most likely diagnosis. Each option may be used once, more than once or not at all.

1. A 32-year-old man presents with sudden-onset shoulder pain after being tackled during a rugby match. On examination, there is loss of the shoulder contour. A mass can be felt in the infraclavicular fossa.
2. A 35-year-old woman presents with an 8-hour history of right shoulder pain that is gradually increasing in severity. There is no history of trauma. The pain is worst on abduction, especially above 120°.
3. A 68-year-old man presents with a 4-month history of shoulder pain that began after he fell over in the park. An X-ray that was performed at the time demonstrated no fracture. Now he complains of pain on all movements of the shoulder. On examination, there is a decreased range of movement, especially external rotation.
4. A 45-year-old man presents with a 2-month history of pain in his left shoulder. The pain is worst in mid-abduction. There is no pain in early or late abduction.
5. A 72-year-old man presented following a fall at home. He is now complaining of shoulder pain. On examination, there is localized tenderness at the acromion and the patient can only minimally abduct this arm. An X-ray of the arm shows no evidence of fracture.

THEME 13: THYROID DISEASE

Options

A. Anaplastic carcinoma
B. de Quervain thyroiditis
C. Follicular carcinoma

D. Graves disease
E. Hashimoto thyroiditis
F. Haemorrhage into a cyst
G. Medullary carcinoma
H. Myxoedema coma
I. Primary myxoedema
J. Thyroid storm
K. Toxic multinodular goitre

For each of the following people with thyroid disease, select the most likely diagnosis. Each option may be used once, more than once or not at all.

1. A 50-year-old woman attends her general practice complaining of low mood and lethargy. She has had this for a few months and has missed much time off work. On further questioning, she admits to being constipated and to having gained weight. On examination, no abnormality is apparent in the neck and no lymphadenopathy is palpable.
2. A 28-year-old woman goes to her general practitioner following a sudden, sharp pain in her neck earlier in the day. Since then, she has found it difficult to breathe. On examination, you find a swelling on the right side of her neck. The patient tells you that this swelling has been there for some time and has never previously caused her any trouble.
3. A 32-year-old woman presents with a 5-week history of resting tremor and diarrhoea. She mentions that just before these symptoms occurred, she had some time off work with a cough and cold. On examination, her pulse is 96/min and regular. The thyroid gland is generally enlarged, soft and tender to touch. No cervical lymph nodes are palpable.
4. A 22-year-old anxious woman presents to her general practitioner with a month's history of worsening diarrhoea. On further questioning, she admits losing 10 pounds over the last few weeks despite having a good appetite. On examination, you notice a slight tremor, and her pulse is 110/min and irregular. Examination of the neck demonstrates no deformity or palpable nodes, although a bruit is heard over the thyroid.
5. A 62-year-old woman is brought by her husband to the emergency department with reduced consciousness. On examination, she has a temperature of 30°C and her pulse is 48/min. Her husband tells you that she has a history of depression and has recently been refusing to take her regular medications.

THEME 14: DIAGNOSIS OF CHEST TRAUMA

Options

A. Abdominal visceral injury
B. Aortic disruption
C. Cardiac tamponade
D. Diaphragmatic rupture

E. Haemothorax
F. Myocardial contusion
G. Open pneumothorax
H. Pulmonary contusion
I. Tension pneumothorax
J. Tracheobrachial injury

For each of the following presentations, select the most likely diagnosis. Each option may be used once, more than once or not at all.

1. A 35-year-old man is involved in a road traffic accident. He was wearing a seatbelt. By the time the paramedics arrive, his blood pressure is 60 mmHg systolic and radial pulses are not palpable. Soon after the cardiac monitor was attached, he went into cardiac arrest.
2. A 35-year-old man is involved in a road traffic accident. He was wearing a seatbelt. By the time the paramedics arrive, he is visibly short of breath, with a respiratory rate of 40/min. On examination, decreased breath sounds are apparent on the left side of the chest, and bowel sounds are audible in the same hemithorax.
3. A 35-year-old man is involved in a road traffic accident. He was wearing a seatbelt. By the time the paramedics arrive, he is sitting by the side of the road attending to a bruise on his left chest. Observations and initial examination are normal, and the patient is admitted for monitoring. A few hours later, he becomes acutely short of breath. An electrocardiogram confirms atrial fibrillation.
4. A 35-year-old man is involved in a road traffic accident. He was wearing a seatbelt. By the time the paramedics arrive, he is complaining of lower left-sided chest and shoulder pain. On examination, his pulse is 132/min and his blood pressure is 90/56 mmHg. Examination of the chest is unremarkable. Despite being given 3 litres of fluid in hospital, the patient is haemodynamically unstable.
5. A 35-year-old man is involved in a road traffic accident. He was wearing a seatbelt. By the time the paramedics arrive, he has managed to walk around, although he has sustained substantial bruising to his chest. Over the next 4 hours he develops worsening respiratory distress. His oxygen saturations are 85% in room air. Percussion and auscultation of the chest are within normal limits, as is an ECG.

THEME 15: ABDOMINAL INCISIONS

Options

A. Battle incision
B. Gridiron incision
C. Kocher incision
D. Lanz incision
E. Midline laparotomy

F. Paramedian incision
G. Pfannenstiel incision
H. Rooftop incision
I. Rutherford Morrison incision
J. Thoracoabdominal incision

For each of the following presentations, select the most appropriate incision to be made. Each option may be used once, more than once or not at all.

1. A 15-year-old girl presents with central abdominal pain that localizes to the right iliac fossa. She also complains of a loss of appetite over the last 24 hours and nausea. On examination, she has a temperature of 37.8°C and is tender in the right iliac fossa.
2. A 40-year-old woman is undergoing elective caesarean section for a breech presentation.
3. A 42-year-old man with known peptic ulcer disease presents with sudden-onset, severe epigastric pain. On examination, he has a tender, rigid abdomen and bowel sounds are absent.
4. A 34-year-old woman is undergoing a laparoscopic cholecystectomy. Unfortunately, the surgeons are unable to clearly delineate the anatomy of the area due to the presence of adhesions.
5. A 64-year-old woman is about to undergo a Whipple procedure for pancreatic adenocarcinoma.

THEME 16: GROIN LUMPS

Options

A. Epididymo-orchitis
B. False femoral aneurysm
C. Mumps orchitis
D. Psoas abscess
E. Saphena varix
F. Sebaceous cyst
G. Strangulated femoral hernia
H. Testicular torsion
I. Testicular tumour

For each of the following people presenting with groin lumps, select the most appropriate diagnosis. Each option may be used once, more than once or not at all.

1. A 22-year-old man presents with a swelling over his medial right thigh. On examination, the swelling is slightly tender and pulsatile but the patient otherwise feels well. The patient admits injecting heroin into the area earlier in the day.
2. An 18-year-old man presents to the emergency department after developing mild pain in the left testicle while playing football. He has no other

symptoms. On examination, the left testicle is larger and more irregular compared with the right.
3. A 28-year-old man presents with a 3-day history of pain in his left testicle. On examination, there is a whitish discharge at the urethral meatus and the scrotum is swollen and tender to palpation.
4. A 37-year-old man presents with a painless swelling in his groin. On examination, the swelling is fluctuant, non-tender and non-pulsatile. The patient does, however, admit to some tenderness in his back. He is currently taking rifampicin and isoniazid for a 'chest infection'.
5. A 13-year-old boy presents with sudden-onset, severe pain in his left testicle, with lower abdominal pain and vomiting. On examination, the testicle is swollen, erythematous and very tender to palpation. The left testicle is lying in the normal position.

THEME 17: MANAGEMENT OF VENOUS DISEASE

Options

A. Elevation, rest and NSAIDs
B. Emergency surgery
C. Injection sclerotherapy
D. Intravenous heparin
E. Reassurance and observation
F. Saphenofemoral ligation
G. Saphenopopliteal ligation
H. Split-skin grafting
I. Subcutaneous low-molecular-weight heparin
J. Systemic antibiotics
K. Topical antibiotics
L. Warfarinization

For each of the following scenarios, select the most appropriate management plan. Each option may be used once, more than once or not at all.

1. A 38-year-old woman who had an elective inguinal hernia repair 6 days ago develops pain in her right calf. On examination, the calf is swollen, tender and erythematous. Pedal pulses are palpable and the patient is otherwise well.
2. A 28-year-old woman was admitted to the ward last night following a paracetamol overdose. She now complains of pain around the cannula site where N-acetylcysteine is being infused. On examination, there is an area of redness adjacent to the cannula and a hard, cord-like structure is palpable under the skin.
3. A 56-year-old woman presents to her general practitioner with a long history of varicose veins. The varicosities are present bilaterally but are asymptomatic and are not troubling the patient.

4. A 64-year-old woman presents with a long history of varicose veins which ache and itch. On examination, she has large varicosities in the distribution of the long saphenous vein. A duplex ultrasound confirms competence of the deep venous system.
5. A 65-year-old woman has a long history of ulceration over her left medial malleolus. Her ABPI is 0.9. She has been managed with compression bandaging for the last 4 months, but there has been no improvement.

Practice Paper 1: Answers

THEME 1: INVESTIGATION OF ABDOMINAL PAIN

1. F – Serum amylase

This man is presenting with features highly suggestive of acute pancreatitis. A markedly raised serum amylase would help confirm this diagnosis quickly. Acute pancreatitis is reversible inflammation of the pancreas. Most cases are caused by gallstones and ethanol. Remember 'GET SMASHED' for the aetiology of acute pancreatitis: Gallstones, Ethanol, Trauma, Steroids, Mumps, Autoimmune, Scorpion venom, Hyperlipidaemia/Hypercalcaemia/Hypothyroidism, Embolism/ERCP, Drugs (azathioprine, steroids, thiazide diuretics and the contraceptive pill). Pregnancy and pancreatic carcinoma are also causes. Many cases of pancreatitis are considered idiopathic in origin. Although scorpion venom is often cited as a cause of acute pancreatitis, it is only the venom of the *Tityus trinitatis* scorpion of Trinidad that has been shown to cause pancreatitis. In fact, scorpion venom is the most common cause of acute pancreatitis in Trinidad.

The pathophysiology of acute pancreatitis is as follows. Duodeno-pancreatic reflux causes duodenal fluid to enter the pancreas and activate the enzymes within it. This results in autodigestion of the pancreas by trypsin, fat necrosis by lipases and a significant rise in circulating amylase. Acute pancreatitis presents with an acute-onset epigastric pain that is severe and constant. It characteristically radiates through to the back and is relieved by sitting forward. Patients may also have nausea and vomiting, fever and features of shock. There may be associated inflammatory exudate and peritonitis, presenting with a distended abdomen and absent bowel sounds. The swollen pancreas can block the distal common bile duct, resulting in jaundice. Inflammatory exudate may collect between the stomach and pancreas, resulting in a pancreatic pseudocyst. This classically presents at day 10 of the disease. Extravasation of blood-stained exudate into the retroperitoneum results in a bluish discolouration of the skin, as the fluid travels between the tissue planes to enter the anterolateral abdominal wall. This can be seen clinically as Cullen sign (periumbilical bruising) and Grey Turner sign (flank bruising).

Plasma amylase levels are increased massively in the acute stage. Mild rises in amylase can occur in many conditions – including trauma, peptic ulcer disease and ruptured aortic aneurysms – and is not specific for pancreatitis. Scoring systems such as the modified Glasgow (Imrie) score are commonly used to indicate disease severity and prognosis.

MODIFIED GLASGOW (IMRIE) SCORING (ONE POINT FOR EACH):

pO_2	<8 KPa
Age	>55 years
Neutrophilia (WCC)	>15 ×10⁹/l
Calcium (corrected)	<2 mmol/l
Raised urea	>16 mmol/l
Enzymes (LDH)	>600 IU/l
Albumin (serum	<32 g/l
Sugar (blood glucose)	>10 mmol/l

Prognosis

1–2 points: <1% mortality
3–4 points: 15% mortality
≥6 points: Mortality rises dramatically towards 100%

Abdominal X-ray may show a single 'sentinel' loop of air-filled bowel next to the pancreas due to localized ileus (or a calcified pancreas if there is a chronic component). A CT scan confirms the diagnosis in the presence of a raised amylase. Management includes opioid analgesia, IV fluids and a proton pump inhibitor. Antibiotics are not indicated unless there is evidence of infection.

Sentinel, from French *sentinelle* = watcher, guard.

Clem Imrie, Emeritus Professor of Surgery, University of Glasgow.

2. B – Erect chest X-ray

It is likely that this woman has perforated an ulcer, which has formed secondary to NSAID use for her osteoarthritis. An erect chest X-ray showing air under the diaphragm will confirm perforation.

3. D – Laparoscopy

This woman could be having another torsion of an ovarian cyst or she could be presenting with appendicitis. A laparoscopy would allow confirmation of the true diagnosis and surgical intervention if required. The management of both appendicitis and twisted ovarian cysts is excision of the lesion. A pelvic ultrasound scan would be a more reasonable next course of action, but this is not one of the options!

Torsion, from Latin *torquere* = to twist.

4. E – Mesenteric angiography

The presentation of severe central abdominal pain that occurs soon after eating is suggestive of mesenteric angina, especially given this patient's history of concurrent atherosclerotic disease in the form of intermittent claudication. An underlying stenosis of the mesenteric arteries would be confirmed by mesenteric angiography.

5. A – CT scan

This man has probably developed an adenocarcinoma of the oesophagus. Chronic reflux into the lower oesophagus can cause the normal squamous cell epithelium to become gastric columnar-type cells. This metaplasia is known as Barrett's oesophagus and is a premalignant condition. Areas of dysplasia can occur in the new epithelium to become adenocarcinoma of the oesophagus in 10%. Most cases occur in the lower third of the oesophagus or at the gastro-oesophageal junction. If adenocarcinoma of the oesophagus is suspected, patients require endoscopy and biopsy followed by a contrast CT scan to verify the spread of disease and to decide whether or not it could be resected.

THEME 2: BURNS

Wallace's 'rule of nines' is a quick way of estimating the surface area involved in burns. The body is divided into units divisible by 9 as follows: 9% for the head and neck, 9% for each upper limb, 18% for the anterior torso, 18% for the posterior torso, 18% for each lower limb, and 1% for the perineum. Another useful tool is that the patient's palm equates to roughly 1% of their body surface area. Only partial and full thickness burns should be included in this calculation. A superficial burn is erythematous and painful without evidence of blistering. It is confined to the epidermis. A second-degree burn (also known as a partial thickness burn) is characteristically red and mottled with evidence of swelling and blistering. Injury extends into the dermis. A third degree burn (full thickness) appears leathery, dry and can be dark or waxy white. It can (but not always) be painless, representing injury to the nerve endings within the subcutaneous layer.

Although the rule of nines is useful for adults, it is not accurate for children due to the relative disproportionate size of certain body parts. Most burns units have charts (such as the Lund and Browder chart) that can more accurately predict body surface areas with respect to age.

1. B – 9%

Right upper limb = 9%

2. F – 27%

Left lower limb + left upper limb = 18% + 9% = 27%

3. F – 27%

Head and neck + anterior torso = 9% + 18% = 27%

4. E – 19%

Right lower limb + perineum = 18% + 1% = 19%

5. H – 37%

Head and neck + right upper limb + left palm + posterior torso = 9% + 9% + 1% + 18% = 37%

Alexander Burns Wallace, Scottish plastic surgeon (1906–1974). Yes, his middle name was 'Burns'!

THEME 3: BACK PAIN

1. D – Posterolateral intervertebral disc herniation

Posterolateral herniation of an intervertebral disc is a common cause of back pain and sciatica. Disc prolapse may be caused by lifting, but is often predisposed to by age-related disc degeneration. The L5/S1 and L4/L5 discs are most commonly affected because these lower discs carry the most weight. Patients present with acute-onset back pain (if the herniation touches the pain-sensitive posterior longitudinal ligament) and sciatica (if a nerve root is involved). The pain diminishes over a few days as the exuded material fibroses and shrinks. On examination, there may be a lumbar scoliosis, reduced flexion and extension (but free lateral flexion) and a restricted straight leg raise on the affected side. Disc protrusion is best seen by MRI and most commonly occurs in the posterior lateral position due to the relative weakness of the posterior longitudinal ligament compared to the thick anterior counterpart (anterior longitudinal ligament). Initial management is with rest, but operative excision of the displaced material can be performed if symptoms are severe or chronic.

A central (posterior) intervertebral disc prolapse at this level will compress the cauda equina, resulting in cauda equina syndrome.

2. I – Spondylosis

Spondylosis is the most common cause of back pain and is considered to be osteoarthritis of the spine. There is initial disc degeneration leading to loss of height with lumbar instability. This results in secondary osteoarthritis of the posterior facet joints. Patients present with an aching pain that is worse on activity and in the mornings. There is a tendency to acute exacerbations of lumbar pain (acute lumbago). On examination, there may be some restriction of spinal movements but no muscle spasm. Management is conservative.

3. F – Spinal stenosis

Spinal stenosis is narrowing of the spinal canal in the lumbar region. The symptoms of spinal stenosis are ascribed to a restriction of the blood supply of the cauda equina in the constricted spinal canal. Affected persons present with back and leg pain on standing and walking. Sitting and bending forwards soon relieves the symptoms because the spinal canal is widened on flexion. The diagnosis is best confirmed by MRI. In severe cases, the spinal canal can be widened surgically.

4. C – Discitis

Discitis is an infection of the intervertebral disc that usually occurs in young children and results in severe pain and a refusal or impairment of mobility. Children are rarely systemically unwell. The cause of discitis is unknown, and treatment is with immobilization with or without antibiotics.

5. G – Spondylolisthesis

Spondylolisthesis is spontaneous displacement of a lumbar vertebral body upon the segment below it. Displacement is usually forwards and occurs at the L4/L5 or L5/S1 level. Spondylolisthesis may be asymptomatic or may result in chronic back pain with sciatica, which is worse on standing. A palpable 'step' of the displaced vertebral body will be felt on examination of the spine. Asymptomatic spondylolisthesis requires no treatment, but severe pain is an indication for surgical release of the affected nerves with fusion of the spinal column.

Spondylolysis is a defect in the neural arch of the fifth lumbar vertebra. There is a loss in the bony continuity between the superior and inferior articular processes, which is instead bridged by fibrous tissue. If this fibrous attachment gives way, it results in spondylolisthesis. Coccydynia is a chronic pain syndrome affecting the coccygeal area that may originate from trauma or childbirth. Pott's disease is tuberculosis infection of the thoracic or lumbar spine, which often results in abscess formation. It presents with pain and stiffness in the back. If an abscess is present, pus can track down the psoas muscle and result in a psoas abscess. Patients with a psoas abscess present with a tender swelling below the inguinal ligament. The affected hip is often held in fixed flexion due to pain.

Percival Pott, English surgeon (1714–1788).

THEME 4: INTESTINAL OBSTRUCTION

The most common causes of small bowel obstruction are (1) adhesions, (2) hernia and (3) tumours. The most common cause of a large bowel obstruction is tumour. When the intestines become obstructed, the bowel distal to the obstruction collapses and the proximal portion dilates. There is increased peristalsis in an attempt to relieve the obstruction, resulting in colic. Eventually, the blood supply to the bowel becomes impaired (ulceration, gangrene and perforation) and pathogens can transudate into the peritoneal cavity (peritonitis). The four cardinal symptoms of intestinal obstruction are colicky abdominal pain + distension + vomiting + obstipation (an inability to pass flatus or faeces). Pain is the first symptom and distension is worse with large bowel obstruction. Vomit contents may be 'faeculent' (not faeces, but instead formed by bacterial decomposition of bowel contents). On examination, tinkling bowel sounds may be heard. Abdominal X-ray confirms dilated loops of bowel in 95% of cases. Treatment of bowel obstruction in general is by drip + suck (IV fluids and nasogastric tube insertion) with or without antibiotics. If conservative therapy fails, the patient proceeds to surgery. Placement of an NG tube serves to decompress the stomach, relieving distention. Patients in obstruction can pool large volumes of fluid in the stomach that can induce vomiting, with a risk of aspiration.

1. I – Sigmoid volvulus

A volvulus is the twisting of a bowel loop around its mesenteric axis. It is most common in the sigmoid or caecum. Risk factors for the development of a volvulus include a long sigmoid, a narrow mesenteric attachment and a constipated loop. Sigmoid volvuli present in older, constipated patients with a sudden-onset abdominal pain. X-ray shows a loop of dilated bowel that twists upon itself ('coffee-bean sign'). Management is by passing a flatus tube into the sigmoid colon via the rectum. If this fails to reduce the volvulus then laparotomy is required. Caecal volvuli are associated with a congenital malformation where the caecum is not fixed to the right iliac fossa. Small bowel volvuli can also occur; these are more common in Africa, and are thought to be due to loading of the small bowel with vegetable matter.

Volvulus, from Latin *volvere* = to roll.

2. A – Adhesions

Adhesions are the most common cause of small bowel intestinal obstruction. Adhesions develop in abdominal cavities that have previously been subject to an operation. The risk of adhesions increases with the number of abdominal surgeries. Therefore patients are at risk of entering a cycle of obstruction followed by laparotomy and adhesiolysis, followed by further adhesions.

3. F – Gallstone ileus

In patients with gallbladder calculi, a stone can erode its way from the gallbladder into the duodenum, forming a cholecysto-duodenal fistula. The stone then passes down the small bowel and lodges in the ileo-caecal junction (the narrowest point distally) resulting in an obstruction. The cholecysto-duodenal fistula then allows air into the biliary tree (a system that is usually air-free). In some cases, a particularly large stone can obstruct the gastric outlet or proximal duodenum by passing through a cholecystogastric or cholecysto-duodenal fistula. This is known as Bouveret syndrome, and is more commonly seen in elderly women with significant co-morbidities. An X-ray will demonstrate air in the biliary tree, dilated small bowel loops and, in some cases, a radio-opaque gallstone in the terminal ileum. Gallstone ileus is a relatively rare cause of small bowel obstruction.

Leon Bouveret, French physician (1850–1929).

4. H – Paralytic ileus

Paralytic ileus is an atonic state of the intestine. The most common cause of a paralytic ileus is postoperative, due to manual handling of the bowel. Other causes of a paralytic ileus are peritonitis, spinal surgery, hypokalaemia, uraemia and anticholinergic drugs. Paralytic ileus presents with vomiting, abdominal distension and absolute constipation. There is an absence of colicky pain as there is no peristalsis. The lack of bowel sounds on auscultation is diagnostic. An abdominal X-ray demonstrates gas in the whole of the small and large bowel, as there is no discrete obstruction. Management is with fluids, NG insertion, pethidine for pain (as it has little effect on GI motility, unlike morphine) and antiemetics. Prolonged paralytic ileus may be treated with metoclopramide, a dopamine antagonist that stimulates gastric emptying and intestine motility. Encouraging the mobilization of patients is also helpful.

5. B – Bezoar

A bezoar is an indigestible mass of material, usually ingested hair or fibres, that is found in the stomach or intestines. It is a rare cause of intestinal obstruction, with a higher incidence among psychiatric or mentally disabled persons. Bezoars are most common in females aged 10–20 years. Endoscopy is required to visualize and remove the lesion. In Medieval times, a bezoar was thought to be a cure for poison (hence the name) – but please don't try this at home!

Bezoar, from Arabic *bazahr* = 'protector from poison'.

THEME 5: ULCERS

1. A – Arterial ulcer

This man has features of intermittent claudication (cramping in the lower limbs on exertion). This is due to underlying ischaemia (from arterial disease). Other features of ischaemia include cold feet, hair loss, toenail dystrophy, dusky cyanosis and ischaemic ulceration. Arterial ulcers are deep, painful and sharply defined, and usually occur on the shin or foot. The peripheral pulses may be reduced or absent on examination. Contrast angiography will help define arterial lesions that may be improved by angioplasty or vascular reconstruction.

2. C – Marjolin ulcer

Marjolin ulcer is the development of a squamous cell carcinoma occurring in an area of scarred or traumatized skin. These include burn injuries, chronic wounds and venous ulcers. Lesions appear as raised, fleshy, firm papules that grow slowly. Treatment is by wide local excision.

Jean-Nicolas Marjolin, French surgeon (1780–1850). He described the condition in 1928.

3. G – Rodent ulcer

A rodent ulcer, or basal cell carcinoma, is a malignant tumour of the basal keratinocytes of the epidermis. It is the most common form of skin cancer, being found typically on the face of middle-aged and older patients with fair skin. Risk factors for the development of rodent ulcers include ultraviolet light exposure, X-ray exposure, chronic scarring, a genetic predisposition and male sex. Lesions classically present as small, skin-coloured papules with telangiectasia and a pearly edge with central necrosis. These tumours grow slowly but relentlessly and are locally invasive, destroying soft tissue, cartilage and bone. Metastasis is very rare. Management is by surgical excision.

4. F – Neuropathic ulcer

This woman with diabetes has developed sensory loss from the ankles distally – in the 'glove-and-stocking' distribution. This neuropathy that occurs with diabetes can result in patients causing severe damage to their feet without noticing, and ulcers can subsequently develop from trivial traumas. For this reason, diabetics should have their peripheral sensation checked regularly, keep their toenails short and avoid walking around barefoot. Neuropathic ulcers often occur on the sole of the foot over areas of pressure (e.g. beneath the metatarsal heads).

5. H – Syphilitic ulcer

The presentation of multiple painless maculopapular ulcers with lymphadenopathy following a primary painless genital ulcer points to a diagnosis of secondary syphilis. Syphilis is a sexually transmitted infection caused by the spirochaete (spiral-shaped) bacterium *Treponema pallidum*. The primary lesion is a single painless ulcer with a clean base (chancre) that occurs at the site of inoculation (i.e. the penis, scrotum, vagina or rectum). A few weeks later, secondary syphilis develops (as above). In some cases, the maculopapular lesions of secondary syphilis can coalesce to form large fleshy masses known as condylomata lata.

Martorell ulcer is an ischaemic ulcer of the leg above the ankle that occurs secondary to hypertension.

Syphilis, from Greek *su* = pig + *philos* = love; 'pig lover'.

Fernando Martorell Otzet, Spanish cardiologist (1906–1984).

THEME 6: MANAGEMENT OF HERNIAS

In order of increasing urgency, the options for managing hernias are observation, elective repair, prompt repair, urgent repair and emergency repair. Elective operations are done at a mutually convenient time. Prompt surgery is surgery that is done early with specific time limits. Urgent operations are done as soon as possible within 24 hours and following adequate resuscitation. Emergency operations are done immediately for life-saving procedures where resuscitation is carried out at the same time as surgery.

1. C – Observation only

This man has a direct inguinal hernia that is reducible and asymptomatic. Hernias that are direct or those that are small and reducible can be managed by observation (unless, of course, it is the patient's wish to have a hernia removed). Patients should have the hernia re-examined after 12 months.

2. B – Emergency repair

This woman presents with a femoral hernia with features of strangulation. As with any painful, irreducible hernia, this should be managed by emergency repair.

3. A – Elective repair

Reducible indirect inguinal hernias are managed by elective operation, as are symptomatic direct inguinal hernias, since these hernias have a relatively low risk of strangulation.

4. E – Urgent repair

This woman has a femoral hernia but has no features of strangulation. Because femoral hernias have a 50% risk of strangulation within 1 month, it is suggested that they should be repaired urgently.

5. D – Prompt repair

This man has an irreducible indirect hernia. Irreducible inguinal hernias, and inguinal hernias that have a history shorter than 4 weeks, should be repaired promptly as there is a greater risk of strangulation in the first 3 months after appearance.

Observe	Direct, reducible, asymptomatic	Re-examine 12 months
Elective repair	Reducible indirect or symptomatic direct	<3% risk of strangulation
Prompt repair	Irreducible indirect or hernia Hx <4/52	Greatest risk of strangulation in first 90 days
Urgent repair	Femoral hernias	50% strangulation risk during first month
Emergency repair	Painful irreducible hernia	

The overwhelming majority of open inguinal hernia procedures utilize the mesh repair. It has a low recurrence rate (1/1000) and the analgesic requirements of patients are low postoperatively.

THEME 7: DIAGNOSIS OF BREAST DISEASE

1. F – Fibrocystic disease

Fibrocystic disease (also known as 'aberrations of normal development and involution') describes disturbances in normal breast physiology. The main pathological abnormalities are small cyst formation, fibrosis and hyperplasia of the duct epithelium. Fibrocystic disease presents with bilateral diffuse lumpiness and breast pain (mastalgia). Clinical features are often cyclical, with increased tenderness and lumpiness just prior to a period, and rapid resolution of symptoms soon after.

2. E – Fibroadenoma

Fibroadenomas are common breast lumps that most frequently occur in women aged 15–25 years. They present as discrete firm, freely mobile lumps, 2–3 cm in size, which classically 'slip' under the examining fingers. For this reason, they are also known as 'breast mice'. Excision of the lesions is not required, as there is no risk of malignancy and most resolve over a period of years.

3. L – Phyllodes tumour

The history of a rapidly growing mass along with the histological findings are typical of a phyllodes tumour. Phyllodes tumours (also known as cystosarcoma phyllodes) are rare tumours of the fibroepithelial stroma of the breast, accounting for <1% of all breast tumours. They are typically benign but fast-growing, and have a distinctive leaf-like appearance on histology (hence the name).

Phyllodes, from Greek *phullon* = leaf.

4. J – Paget disease

Paget disease of the nipple is an eczema-like (i.e. dry and itchy) condition of the nipple that persists despite local treatment and is associated with an underlying breast carcinoma. As the disease progresses, the nipple erodes and eventually disappears. The diagnosis of Paget disease is confirmed by biopsy of the lesion.

Sir James Paget, English surgeon (1814–1899).

5. K – Peau d'orange

Peau d'orange describes a characteristic appearance of the breast that can occur in association with breast cancer. There is cutaneous lymphoedema with dimpling where the skin is tethered by sweat ducts that have been infiltrated with cancer.

Peau d'orange, from French, *peau* = skin; 'orange-skin'.

Duct ectasia is a benign condition of the breast characterized by enlargement of the ducts within the subareolar region, with eosinophilic granular secretions and foamy histiocytes detected on microscopic analysis. Fat necrosis is seen following breast trauma. The injured adipose tissue can harden into scar tissue or develop into an oil cyst. Investigation is by means of triple assessment. A galactocele (or lactocele) is another benign breast condition characterized by a retention cyst resulting from lactiferous duct occlusion. Gynaecomastia is the development of breast tissue in men and is the result of excess circulating oestrogens.

Prolactinomas are the most common type of pituitary tumour accounting for up to 30% of cases. Prolactinomas are five times more common in women, but males tend to develop macroadenomas more frequently. Symptoms include infertility, gynaecomastia, galactorrhea (inappropriate milk production) and reduced libido.

THEME 8: MANAGEMENT OF TESTICULAR CONDITIONS

1. D – Excision of cyst

The presentation of a tense, smooth, fluctuant, transilluminating swelling around the testicle suggests a hydrocele. This patient should have a testicular ultrasound to exclude an underlying cause for the swelling, such as malignancy. Management of primary hydroceles is by excision of the cyst. Simple aspiration of the cysts risks introducing infection into the testicle, and aspirated cysts have a high incidence of recurrence.

2. L – Reduction and fixation

This patient presents with features of testicular torsion, where twisting of the spermatic cord results in ischaemia of the testicle. Testicular torsion is an acute surgical emergency and requires surgical exploration within 6 hours to reduce and fix the testis before necrosis occurs.

3. H – Orchidectomy + radiotherapy

The presence of an irregular painless testicular lump is indicative of testicular cancer. There are two main types of testicular cancer: seminomas (60%) and teratomas (40%). Seminomas arise from the seminiferous tubules and occur in the 30–40-year age group. Teratomas arise from germ cells and occur in the 20–30-year age group. Considering this patient's age, he is more likely to have a seminoma. Remember Sergeants (Seminomas) and Troops (Teratomas).

All testicular tumours – seminomas and teratomas – are managed by radical inguinal orchidectomy. Further treatment depends on the type of tumour and the presence of nodal metastases (which is elicited by staging CT scans). Seminomas that have no evidence of spread (as in this scenario) or that have only small nodal metastases are managed by orchidectomy and radiotherapy to the para-aortic lymph nodes to reduce recurrence. If there is extensive nodal metastatic spread then combination chemotherapy is added.

4. A – Antibiotics

This man presents with epididymo-orchitis, which has probably occurred secondary to urethritis (dysuria and pyuria). Epididymo-orchitis tends to be caused by enteric flora in older men (usually *Escherichia coli*), but is commonly caused by sexually transmitted infections (*Chlamydia trachomatis* and *Neisseria gonorrhoea*) in men under the age of 35 years. Management is with bed rest, scrotal support and appropriate empirical antibiotics, such as ciprofloxacin and doxycyline. The presentation of torsion is similar, and if this cannot be confidently excluded then surgical exploration is required.

5. G – Orchidectomy + chemotherapy

This man has a teratoma with evidence of lymphatic spread. Unlike seminomas, teratomas are not radiosensitive, so metastatic disease is managed with orchidectomy and combination chemotherapy. Teratomas that show no evidence of spread are treated by orchidectomy alone and surveillance.

Germ cell tumours can be benign or malignant. They are classified into seminomatous germ cell tumours (SGCT) and non-seminomatous germ cell tumours (NSGCT). NSGCTs include teratomas and choriocarcinomas. This histological distinction is made because of the important distinction in treatment. Seminomas are highly radiosensitive and respond well to chemotherapy. NSGCTs are insensitive to radiotherapy, grow faster and carry a poorer prognosis.

THEME 9: HYPERSENSITIVITY REACTIONS

Hypersensitivity reactions are classified using the Gell and Coombs system as follows:

Type I (anaphylactic)	IgE-mediated from allergen exposure
Type II (cytotoxic)	Antibody-mediated
Type III	Immune complex-mediated
Type IV (delayed)	Sensitized T-cell-mediated
Type V (stimulatory)	Stimulatory anti-receptor antibody-mediated

Robin Coombs, British immunologist (1921–2006).
Philip Gell, British immunologist (1914–2001).

1. A – Type I hypersensitivity

Type I hypersensitivity (anaphylactic) reactions occur when exposure to certain allergens results in IgE-mediated secretion of inflammatory mediators by basophils and mast cells. The linkage of two IgE molecules by an antigen results in the release of inflammatory mediators, such as histamine and prostaglandins. This results in vasodilation and smooth muscle contraction, and symptoms range from mild irritation to anaphylactic shock and death. Treatment is with adrenaline, antihistamines (chlorphenamine) and steroids. Examples of type I hypersensitivity reactions include allergic asthma, atopic eczema, hay fever (allergic rhinitis) and peanut allergies.

2. C – Type III hypersensitivity

Type III hypersensitivity reactions are mediated by immune complexes (antigen-antibody complexes). Immune complexes can deposit in various sites in the body and result in localized tissue damage via complement activation. Complexes can also form thrombi and induce tissue ischaemia. Small complexes are filtered by the glomeruli whilst large ones are destroyed by macrophages. An example of immune complex damage is glomerulonephritis following a streptococcal throat infection, as in this case. Other examples of type III hypersensitivity reactions include rheumatic fever and systemic lupus erythematosus.

3. E – Type V hypersensitivity

Type V (stimulatory) hypersensitivity reactions describe the presence of antibodies that bind to cell receptors and either stimulate or prevent stimulation of the receptor. Examples include Graves disease (this scenario – a stimulatory response of autoantibodies binding to the TSH receptor of the thyroid gland) and myasthenia gravis (an inhibitory response from autoantibodies that bind to acetylcholine receptors at the neuromuscular junction).

4. D – Type IV hypersensitivity

Type IV hypersensitivity reactions are known as delayed-type reactions as features can take days to develop. T cells can become sensitized by certain allergens, and this results in cytotoxic T-cell-mediated cell damage. Examples of type IV hypersensitivity reactions include contact dermatitis (e.g. to nickel or beryllium) and transplant rejection.

5. B – Type II hypersensitivity

In type II hypersensitivity reactions, autoantibodies bind to the cell surfaces (as opposed to cell receptors as in type V reactions). This results in autoantibody-mediated destruction of cells. Examples of type II hypersensitivity reactions include haemolytic disease of the newborn (this scenario), transfusion reactions and autoimmune thrombocytopenia.

THEME 10: NECK LUMPS

1. D – Cystic hygroma

A cystic hygroma is a congenital benign proliferation of lymph vessels that is found in the posterior triangle of the neck. It is a multicystic swelling that is fleshy and compressible and contains clear fluid. Cystic hygromas characteristically transilluminate 'brightly'. Diagnosis is confirmed by CT or MRI, and treatment is by excision of the mass.

Hygroma, from Greek *hygros* = wet + *oma* = tumour; so-called as it contains fluid.

The posterior triangle of the neck is bounded by the sternocleidomastoid muscle in front, the anterior border of the trapezius behind and the middle third of the clavicle at its base. The apex of the triangle is the occiput.

2. F – Salivary duct carcinoma

Salivary duct carcinoma is an aggressive tumour that occurs in the over-50 age group. There is a rapidly growing, infiltrating mass associated with regional node involvement and rapid metastasis. The facial nerve, which passes through the parotid gland, is often involved (unlike the benign pleomorphic adenoma) and this can result in unilateral weakness of the facial muscles. Treatment is by radical parotidectomy (including excision of the facial nerve), but the prognosis is still poor.

3. B – Branchial cyst

A branchial cyst occurs secondary to cystic degeneration of lymphoid tissue. It is more common in males on the left side. Branchial cysts are smooth, non-tender, fluctuant swellings in the anterior triangle, anterior to the border of the sternocleidomastoid muscle at the junction of its upper and middle thirds. Unlike cystic hygromas, they do not transilluminate. Branchial cysts may become enlarged and tender with upper respiratory tract infections. Diagnosis is by aspiration, which demonstrates a creamy fluid that contains cholesterol crystals. Treatment is by excision.

4. I – Thyroglossal cyst

A thyroglossal cyst is a congenital cystic remnant of the thyroglossal tract. It usually presents in the first decade as a smooth midline lump that moves up on tongue protrusion (note that thyroid lumps do not move up with protrusion of the tongue). Diagnosis is by ultrasound, and treatment is by excision of the cyst and thyroglossal duct (Sistrunk operation).

Thyroglossal, from Greek *thyreoeides* = shield-shaped + *glossus* = tongue; the thyroid was thought of as the shield-shaped gland.

Walter Sistrunk, American surgeon (1880–1933).

5. G – Salivary gland stone

Salivary gland stones (sialolithiasis) are made of calcium and result in blockage of the salivary ducts. Features include immense pain on salivation, with associated enlargement of the gland. Plain X-ray may show larger stones, but the best way to demonstrate stenosis or blockage of the salivary ducts is by sialography, where radioactive contrast is injected into the duct system. Management may require removal of the offending gland. In sialolithiasis, the blockage of saliva predisposes to bacterial infection of the gland. This condition is known as acute bacterial sialolithiasis.

Sialolithiasis, from Greek *sialon* = saliva + *lith* = stone.

Acute bacterial sialolithiasis is a bacterial infection of the salivary gland most likely secondary to an occluding stone. The submandibular gland and its associated duct (Wharton duct) is the most likely to be affected. The examining clinician should look for discharging pus from the exit of the gland under a small papillae either side of the lingual frenulum. Chemodectoma is a rare neuroendocrine tumour of the chemoreceptors of the carotid bodies and the aortic arch. Virchow node is an eponymous unilateral lymph node found in the left supraclavicuar fossa. Its presence is associated with breast and intra-abdominal malignancy.

Rudolph Virchow, German pathologist (1821–1902).

THEME 11: CLASSIFICATION OF JAUNDICE

Jaundice is defined as an elevation of serum bilirubin. The metabolism of bilirubin is as follows. The haem components of red blood cells are broken down by macrophages in the spleen and bone marrow to produce unconjugated bilirubin. This unconjugated bilirubin is insoluble and therefore not excretable. It is transported to the liver bound to albumin where hepatocytes conjugate the bilirubin with glucoronide, making it soluble so that it can be excreted via the biliary tract into the duodenum. Duodenal bilirubin travels to the terminal ileum, where it is converted into urobilinogen. Urobilinogen has three fates: it can be absorbed by the blood and excreted via the kidneys into urine; it can be converted to stercobilinogen and excreted with faeces; or it can be reabsorbed and re-excreted by the liver (hepatic recycling).

Jaundice, from Latin *galbinus* = yellowish-green, via the Old French *jaunisse.*

The causes of jaundice are divided into pre-hepatic, hepatic and post-hepatic, depending on where the underlying abnormality is. Pre-hepatic jaundice results from an increased bile production due to haemolysis. Examples include hereditary spherocytosis and haemolytic transfusion reactions. These cause an unconjugated (insoluble) hyperbilirubinaemia, so no bilirubin is found in the urine. Hepatic jaundice is due to impaired bile conjugation and excretion in the liver, for example with hepatitis, cirrhosis, drugs and tumours. In this case there is a mixed unconjugated and conjugated hyperbilirubinaemia. Post-hepatic jaundice is caused by biliary obstruction, for example by gallstones, tumour or infection. This results in a conjugated (soluble) hyperbilirubinaemia with pale stools and dark urine. The investigation of the jaundiced patient should include a full blood count, clotting studies, CRP, ESR, auto-antibodies and virology.

1. B – Hepatic

An isolated hyperbilirubinaemia in an asymptomatic patient is indicative of Gilbert syndrome. Because this condition involves a defect in bilirubin conjugation, it is a cause of hepatic jaundice.

Augustin Nicholas Gilbert, French physician (1858–1927).

2. B – Hepatic

Both rifampicin and isoniazid are known to cause hepatitis, and therefore hepatic jaundice. Other drugs that are known to cause hepatitis include allopurinol, amitriptyline, amiodarone, ibuprofen, halothane and phenytoin. Statins can cause deranged liver function tests without any underlying hepatitis.

3. A – Pre-hepatic

This woman is suffering from a transfusion-related haemolytic reaction. The increased breakdown of red cells results in a massive rise in unconjugated bilirubin; hence it is a pre-hepatic jaundice. No bilirubin is found in the urine as the unconjugated bilirubin is tightly bound to albumin and unable to pass through the glomerulus.

4. C – Post-hepatic

The presence of pale stools and dark urine indicates an element of conjugated (soluble) hyperbilirubinaemia. The history suggests a stone in the common bile duct – a post-hepatic cause of jaundice. Dark urine is seen because of the increased urobilinogen. The pale stools result from low levels of stercobilinogen (as the obstructed biliary tree prevents bilirubin from passing into the intestinal tract). Both dark stools and pale urine are consequences of impaired bile excretion into the GI tract.

5. B – Hepatic

This man is showing symptoms of acute viral hepatitis. Because it affects the liver itself, it is another hepatic cause of jaundice.

THEME 12: SHOULDER DISORDERS

1. A – Anterior dislocation

Anterior dislocation of the shoulder is usually caused by a fall on the outstretched hand or onto the shoulder itself. It presents with severe shoulder pain and an unwillingness to move the arm. The contour of the shoulder is flattened so the acromion process is the most lateral point of the shoulder region. The humeral head may be palpable in the infraclavicular fossa. Various manoeuvres are available to help reduce dislocated shoulders. The axillary nerve is damaged in 5% of anterior dislocations, and it is important to document neurovascular status before reducing any dislocation. After an initial anterior dislocation, part of the joint capsule is stripped from the scapula (the Bankart lesion). This creates an intracapsular pocket into which recurrent dislocations can occur when the arm is in lateral rotation, abduction and extension (such as when putting on a coat).

Posterior dislocation accounts for only 2% of shoulder dislocations. It is usually due to an electric shock, an epileptic fit or a direct blow to the front of the shoulder. There is fixed medial rotation of the arm with anterior flattening of the normal contour below the acromion. Diagnosis is confirmed by a lateral X-ray.

2. G – Supraspinatus tendonitis

Acute calcific tendonitis of the supraspinatus tendon usually occurs in younger women. Deposition of calcium hydroxyapatite crystals on the medial insertion of the supraspinatus tendon results in acute-onset severe shoulder pain. The pain is worst on abduction above 120° – this is different to the range of maximal pain in the impingement syndrome (see below). The pain worsens over a few hours and gradually subsides over a few days.

3. B – Frozen shoulder

Frozen shoulder (also known as adhesive capsulitis) is a relatively common condition and frequently follows a history of minor trauma in middle-aged adults. Patients present with a long history of aching pain and restriction of all gleno-humeral movements (flexion, extension, rotation and abduction). External rotation is the first movement to be restricted. Spontaneous recovery takes place over 12–24 months. Physiotherapy and steroid injections may help aid recovery. The natural course of the disease follows three characteristic phases: freezing, frozen and thawing. The 'freezing' phase is characterized principally by pain, with increasing stiffness. Pain eases during the 'frozen' stage at the expense of a reduction in movement. Both pain and stiffness improve whilst the shoulder 'thaws'.

4. C – Impingement syndrome

In the impingement syndrome (also known as painful arc syndrome) there is pain on abduction between 60° and 120° only. The pain is produced by mechanical nipping of a tender structure between the greater tuberosity of the humerus and the acromion process. The primary lesions that give rise to the painful arc syndrome are incomplete tear of the supraspinatus, chronic supraspinatus tendonitis, subacromial bursitis and a crack fracture of the greater tuberosity.

5. E – Rotator cuff tear

The rotator cuff is a ring of muscles and tendons that provide stability to the shoulder girdle. It is made up of four muscles (supraspinatus, infraspinatus, subscapularis and teres minor). Rotator cuff tears typically occur in older patients following trauma and usually involve the supraspinatus tendon. The most common site of the tear is the 'critical zone' of the supraspinatus tendon, a relatively avascular region near its insertion. Patients present with shoulder tip pain and an inability to abduct the arm. There is localized tenderness at the lateral margin of the acromion. If the arm is abducted to above 90° with assistance then the patient can sustain the abduction by action of the deltoid muscle (the 'abduction paradox'). If the arm is lowered below 90°, it suddenly drops (the 'drop arm' sign).

The long tendon of the biceps muscle is prone to rupture in older people without violent stress or injury due to underlying age-related degeneration. It occurs commonly in middle-aged men, who feel moderate discomfort of the arm whilst lifting. On examination, there is slight tenderness in the bicipital groove and an unusual bulge is seen on elbow flexion. Surprisingly, there is only a slight weakness of flexion and supination.

THEME 13: THYROID DISEASE

1. I – Primary myxoedema

The woman in this question presents with some classic features of an underactive thyroid. This, along with the lack of goitre, makes primary myxoedema the best answer. Primary myxoedema is also known as spontaneous atrophic hypothyroidism. It is characterized by an idiopathic reduction in the production of thyroid hormones. Features of hypothyroidism include a hoarse voice, constipation, feeling cold, weight gain, low mood, lethargy, coarse hair and dysmenorrhoea. The diagnosis of primary hypothyroidism is made by demonstrating a low T4 (thyroxine) despite a high TSH (thyroid-stimulating hormone). Hypothyroidism is treated with daily thyroxine, which is taken for life.

Myxoedema, from Greek *myxa* = slime + *oedema* = swelling.

2. F – Haemorrhage into a cyst

The woman in this case has a history of a thyroid cyst. The acute presentation of neck pain and growth of the lesion suggests haemorrhage into the cyst. Haemorrhage can result in tracheal compression and stridor. If possible, aspiration of the cyst contents should be performed to alleviate tracheal compression and maintain airway patency. If aspiration is not possible, surgical intervention may be required.

3. B – de Quervain thyroiditis

de Quervain thyroiditis (or 'subacute thyroiditis') is usually precipitated by a viral infection, such as influenza, coxsackievirus or mumps. There is inflammation of the thyroid gland, with subsequent release of thyroid hormones, resulting in a transient mild hyperthyroidism (hence the tremor and diarrhoea in this patient). Patients present with pain in the thyroid region, neck, jaw and ears that is worse with swallowing and neck movement. Eventually, the thyroid function returns to normal, although some patients become mildly hypothyroid for up to 6 months. de Quervain thyroiditis requires no specific treatment, but non-steroidal anti-inflammatories can be given for pain.

Fritz de Quervain, Swiss surgeon (1868–1940).

4. D – Graves disease

This woman demonstrates features of thyrotoxicosis (anxiety, diarrhoea, tremor and weight loss despite a good appetite) with a thyroid bruit. The presence of hyperthyroidism with a bruit indicates a likely diagnosis of Graves disease. Graves disease is an autoimmune condition resulting in overactivity of the thyroid. The hyperthyroidism is due to the presence of antibodies that stimulate the TSH receptor, resulting in a high secretion of thyroid hormones. Apart from the generic features of thyrotoxicosis (such as diarrhoea, feeling warm, weight loss despite a good appetite, tremor), patients with Graves disease may also demonstrate a thyroid bruit (which occurs secondary to hyperdynamic flow), pretibial myxoedema and ophthalmoplegia. Specific examples of eye disease in Graves disease are lid retraction and proptosis (a 'bulging' appearance of the eyes due to myxoedematous infiltration of the muscles behind the eye). Treatment options for hyperthyroidism include carbimazole, iodine-131 and subtotal thyroidectomy. Beta-blockers, such as propranolol, help diminish the symptoms of thyrotoxicosis but do not affect the underlying disease.

Robert James Graves, Irish physician (1797–1853).

5. H – Myxoedema coma

Older patients with undiagnosed hypothyroidism, or those who do not take their medications, can present with features of severe hypothyroidism, or a myxoedema coma. These include impaired consciousness, hypothermia, bradycardia and hypoglycaemia. The woman in this scenario has this presentation, and it could be that her regular medication included thyroxine for hypothyroidism (which could have caused her depression). Patients with a myxoedema coma should be transferred to intensive care for fluids, gentle rewarming and intravenous thyroid hormones. The mortality rate is 50%.

The opposite condition, where there is a sudden large concentration of circulating thyroid hormones, is called a 'thyroid storm'. It can be precipitated by infection or stress. Patients present with fever, tachycardia, agitation, atrial fibrillation and heart failure. Treatment is again in intensive care with fluids, gentle cooling and intravenous beta-blockers (propranolol). Sodium iopodate (which inhibits thyroxine release) and carbimazole (inhibits synthesis of thyroxine) are also administered. The mortality rate is around 10%.

There are four principle types of thyroid cancer: papillary, follicular, medullary and anaplastic. Papillary is the most common type accounting for up to 80% of cases. Histological analysis demonstrates a characteristic 'Orphan Annie eye' appearance nuclei (nuclei which appear empty and demonstrate uniform staining). It has a 5-year survival of 90%. Follicular carcinoma is the second most common representing 15% of thyroid cancers. Formal diagnosis is made if capsular invasion is seen or invasion of the vasculature around the tumour periphery. Survival is 70% at 5 years. Medullary carcinoma is associated with multiple endocrine neoplasia (MEN) II. It is a cancer of the calcitonin-secreting parafollicular C cells which, when stained with Congo red, demonstrates characteristic apple-green birefringence. Medullary carcinoma accounts for approximately 8% of thyroid cancer and carries a survival of 60% at 5 years. Anaplastic thyroid cancer carries the worst prognosis with virtually no one surviving more than 5 years following diagnosis. Thankfully, it is also the rarest form representing fewer than 5% of thyroid cancers. It is more common in the elderly.

One method of remembering the route of spread of thyroid cancers is as follows:

Papillary	Yellow	Lymph
Follicular	Red	Blood
Medullary	Yellow	Lymph
Anaplastic	Combined	Lymph and blood

THEME 14: DIAGNOSIS OF CHEST TRAUMA

1. B – Aortic disruption

Aortic disruption occurs with a rapid deceleration injury, and the site of rupture is often the ligamentum arteriosum, as this is where the mobile aortic arch is anchored. Other deceleration injuries are likely to occur wherever a mobile structure links with a fixed one (the brain inside the cranial vault is another example). The massive hypovolaemia in this man, as suggested by the profound hypotension and lack of radial pulses, are signs of disruption or dissection of the aorta. The majority (90%) of these injuries are immediately fatal. A chest X-ray in aortic dissection/disruption will show a widened mediastinum, and a spiral CT scan with contrast will confirm the diagnosis. Immediate management of aortic disruption is by fluid resuscitation to maintain the blood pressure, but definitive surgical intervention is required.

2. D – Diaphragmatic rupture

Diaphragmatic injuries are rare and can occur as a result of blunt trauma that causes a massive pressure gradient between the peritoneal and pleural cavities. Over 80% of diaphragmatic ruptures occur on the left side, as the liver is protective on the right. The tears in the diaphragm usually occur at the posterolateral aspect, the embryological weak point. Following diaphragmatic rupture, the abdominal contents herniate into the thorax. Features therefore include respiratory compromise. On examination, there may be tracheal deviation away from the side of injury. Breath sounds and chest expansion will also be reduced unilaterally. Bowel sound may be heard loudly in the affected hemithorax. A chest X-ray will show herniated abdominal contents in the thorax. If diagnosis is in doubt, a CT scan +/– contrast studies can be performed. After initial resuscitation, treatment is by surgical repair of the rupture.

3. F – Myocardial contusion

Blunt trauma to the chest can result in damage to the myocardium, cardiac chamber or valves. Myocardial contusion is a bruising of the cardiac muscle. Initially, patients are aware only of chest wall bruising or fractures. The features of myocardial contusion only occur later on, presenting as hypotension and ECG abnormalities such as sinus tachycardia, atrial fibrillation, bundle branch block and ST segment changes. Patients diagnosed with myocardial contusion require cardiac monitoring for at least 24 hours because they are at risk of sudden dysrhythmias.

4. A – Abdominal visceral injury

This man has a lower left-sided injury with refractory hypotension. It is likely that he has ruptured his spleen. The spleen is one of the most commonly injured abdominal viscera, often following trauma to the abdomen or lower left ribs. Features of splenic rupture include those of haemorrhage shock (hypotension, tachycardia and peripheral vasoconstriction), abdominal pain and distension, and referred pain to the left shoulder tip secondary to diaphragmatic irritation by intraperitoneal blood (Kehr sign). Investigation of a suspected ruptured spleen depends on the haemodynamic status of the patient. Stable patients can undergo CT, whereas unstable patients require urgent laparotomy. If there are no signs of progressive haemorrhage, splenic ruptures can be managed conservatively with observation for 7–10 days. Otherwise splenectomy is required.

Splenic injuries can be classified into grades I to V according to the American Association for the Surgery of Trauma, as follows:

Grade I: Subcapsular haematoma (capsular laceration <1 cm)
Grade II: Subcapsular haematoma 10–50% of surface area, intraparenchymal haematoma <5 cm in diameter
Grade III: Subcapsular haematoma >50% of surface area, or intraparenchymal haematoma >5 cm in diameter
Grade IV: Laceration involving hilar or segmental vessels
Grade V: Shattered spleen

It is important to be aware of post-splenectomy prophylaxis. All patients who have had a splenectomy should be made aware of the risks and carry an 'I've had a splenectomy!' card with them. They will also require vaccinations for the three main encapsulated organisms that are usually destroyed by the spleen *(Streptococcus pneumoniae, Haemophilus influenzae B* and *Neisseria meningitides),* with boosters at 10 years. Prophylactic antibiotics are not necessarily required lifelong, but only till the age of 15 years. The drug of choice is amoxicillin (or erythromycin to those who are penicillin-allergic). Patients should, however, be provided with antibiotics for any febrile illness.

5. H – Pulmonary contusion

Bruising to the lung is a potentially fatal chest injury and can occur following blunt trauma. Most cases are associated with multiple rib fractures or a flail chest. Initial observations may be normal, but features of respiratory failure develop insidiously due to increasing airway resistance and decreased compliance of the affected lung. Management is with respiratory support and analgesia. Patients with significant hypoxia (oxygen saturations <90% or pO_2 <8.0 kPa) or underlying chronic lung disease will require intubation and ventilation.

THEME 15: ABDOMINAL INCISIONS

Ideally, abdominal incisions will allow ready access to the relevant organs and may be extended easily. There should be a good cosmetic outcome and patients should be left relatively pain-free postoperatively. Langer's lines mark the principle axis of orientation of the collagen fibres of the dermis and form the natural creases of the skin. Incisions that are made parallel to these lines offer the best cosmetic outcome.

1. D – Lanz incision

This young girl presents with appendicitis. There are two abdominal incisions available for an open appendicectomy: the gridiron and Lanz incisions. The gridiron incision is made one-third of the way along, and at right angles to, the line connecting the anterior superior iliac spine to the umbilicus in the right iliac fossa (i.e. McBurney's point). It is generally the incision of choice for an open appendicectomy. A Lanz incision is more transverse in orientation and closer to the anterior superior iliac spine when compared to the gridiron incision, and is made in the skin crease. A Lanz incision is preferred in younger females as it provides a better cosmetic result. However, these incisions tend to divide the iliohypogastric and ilioinguinal nerves, resulting in denervation of the muscles of the inguinal canal, increasing the risk of inguinal hernia. An alternative option here would be laparoscopy. The advantage being other causes of the patient's symptoms could be investigated should the appendix be macroscopically normal (such as torsion of an ovarian cyst or inflammatory bowel disease). Should there be a high suspicion of appendicitis (i.e. confirmed by CT scan) one can argue an open appendicectomy can result in less scarring than laparoscopy.

Otto Lanz, Swiss surgeon (1865–1935).

2. G – Pfannenstiel incision

Pfannenstiel incision is a transverse incision made 5 cm above the pubic symphysis and around 10–12 cm across in the midline. It is used commonly by gynaecologists (for caesarean sections and ovarian operations) and urologists (for access to the bladder and prostate). Pfannenstiel incision offers excellent cosmetic results.

Hans Hermann Johannes Pfannenstiel, German gynaecologist (1862–1909).

3. E – Midline laparotomy

This presentation is suggestive of a perforated peptic ulcer, which will require surgical intervention. An incision needs to be made that is quick and allows easy access to the gut, and a midline laparotomy is the most suitable. A midline incision is made through the linea alba. This is a relatively avascular incision that can be made, extended and closed easily. Incisions cross Langer's lines and thus are cosmetically poor. The incision also crosses multiple dermatomes (T7–T12 should it be a full-length incision) so good postoperative pain control is required.

4. C – Kocher incision

Kocher incision is made 3 cm below and parallel to the subcostal margin from the midline to the border of the rectus abdominus muscle. A right-sided Kocher incision is appropriate for an open cholecystectomy. Left-sided incisions are used for splenectomy. The incision cannot be extended medially and, if it is extended too far laterally, many intercostal nerves can be damaged.

Emil Theodore Kocher, Swiss surgeon (1841–1917).

5. H – Rooftop incision

A rooftop incision (or double Kocher incision) is made up of both a left and a right Kocher's incision connected at the middle. It provides good access to the liver and spleen. It is also indicated for use in bilateral adrenalectomy and for radical pancreatic and gastric surgery.

Battle's incision was a vertical incision made just medial to the lateral border of the abdominal rectus muscle. It was previously used for appendicitis, but is no longer recommended, as it damages nerves entering the rectus sheath and has a high risk of incisional hernia. Paramedian incisions are made 1.5 cm from the midline through the rectus sheath. They were popular in the days when suture materials were not as good, but are avoided now due to the poor cosmetic result. A Rutherford Morrison incision is an extended version of the gridiron incision that allows good views of the caecum and right colon. Thoraco-abdominal incisions allow access to the lower thorax and upper abdomen.

William Henry Battle, English surgeon (1855–1936).

James Rutherford Morrison, British surgeon (1853–1939).

THEME 16: GROIN LUMPS

1. B – False femoral aneurysm

A false aneurysm (or pseudoaneurysm) is one that does not involve the vessel wall (unlike a true aneurysm, which involves all three layers of the blood vessel – namely the intima, media and adventitia). It represents an accumulation of blood (haematoma) that is held in proximity to the vessel by the surrounding connective tissue. False aneurysm may follow traumatic damage to an artery, such as in femoral artery cannulation for angiography or after incorrect placement of needles by intravenous drug users. False aneurysms of the femoral artery present as expansile pulsatile masses in the groin with a history of trauma to the region. Small pseudoaneurysms will clot spontaneously, whereas larger ones will need surgical intervention.

2. I – Testicular tumour

Testicular tumours are the most common solid tumours in young adult males. They can present with a testicular lump, a secondary hydrocele or testicular pain. Do not be fooled by the pain occurring on activity – a hard, irregular testicle should be considered cancer until proven otherwise. An urgent ultrasound scan should therefore be arranged. For notes regarding testicular tumours see Answers to Paper 1, Theme 8.

3. A – Epididymo-orchitis

Epididymo-orchitis (inflammation of the epididymis and testis) presents with a painful swelling of the epididymis with constitutional symptoms, such as pyrexia and malaise. Patients may also exhibit a secondary hydrocele. Because epididymo-orchitis is usually a consequence of ascending infection (e.g. from a urinary tract infection or a sexually transmitted urethritis), there may also be a history of dysuria or urethral discharge. When someone presents with a painful, swollen testicle, it is important to rule out testicular torsion – if in doubt, the patient should be referred for urgent surgical exploration. Treatment of epididymo-orchitis is with bed rest and a long course of antibiotics (e.g. 6 weeks of oral ciprofloxacin). If an abscess develops, it requires drainage.

4. D – Psoas abscess

This man is taking rifampicin and isoniazid – antimicrobial drugs used to treat tuberculosis infection. A recognized complication of tuberculosis is the development of a paraspinal abscess (Pott disease). If this abscess tracks down the psoas muscle towards the groin, an inguinal psoas abscess can arise. A psoas abscess is usually fluctuant, painless and not warm (hence it is given the term 'cold abscess', which is characteristic of tuberculosis infection). Pain is exacerbated by contraction or extension of the psoas muscle (the principle hip flexor). The diagnosis of a psoas abscess is best made by MRI and confirmed on Gram and acid fast bacilli (AFB) staining and culture of aspirated fluid.

Percival Pott, British surgeon (1714–1788).

5. H – Testicular torsion

The development of sudden-onset pain and swelling in the testicle strongly suggests torsion of the testicle, which is a surgical emergency. Patients may also suffer referred pain in the lower abdomen and groin (due to the T10 nerve, which supplies the lower abdomen as well as the testes) along with nausea and vomiting. The torsion occurs around the spermatic cord when there is an anatomically abnormal testicle, often following a history of mild trauma. An example of an anatomical anomaly is the 'bell-clapper' testis, where the testicle is not anchored to the scrotum posteriorly by gubernaculum ligament (as it should be normally), leaving it to swing freely like the clapper of a bell.

In testicular torsion, the testis may be riding high within the scrotum, although a normal lie of the testicle does not exclude torsion. (The left testicle normally hangs lower than the right.) Irreversible infarction of a twisted testicle occurs within 6–12 hours, so affected patients should be taken to theatre for surgical exploration without further investigation. Surgical management includes untwisting of the testicle following a midline scrotal incision and watching it 'pink up' (revascularize). Bilateral fixation (orchidopexy) of the testes to the tunica vaginalis is required to prevent further torsion. This is necessary because the anatomical abnormalities of the testes that predispose to torsion usually occur on both sides.

THEME 17: MANAGEMENT OF VENOUS DISEASE

1. I – Subcutaneous low-molecular-weight heparin

This woman has developed a postoperative deep vein thrombosis. Management can either be with intravenous heparin or subcutaneous low-molecular-weight heparins (LMWHs). Heparin requires a loading dose followed by a continuous infusion, and the dose of the drug is modified according to daily measurements of activated partial thromboplastin time (APTT). LMWHs are much easier to administer (once-daily injection) and do not require monitoring. For this reason, LMWH is the first-line treatment for deep vein thrombosis and pulmonary embolism. Heparin is reserved for patients with severe, life-threatening thromboembolism. Treatment with LMWHs or heparin is continued for 7 days, followed by warfarinization. Warfarin should not be given immediately because it has a pro-thrombotic effect when first given (due to an inhibition of the antithrombotic proteins C and S) and it can take several days before therapeutic levels are reached. In life-threatening pulmonary embolism, thrombolytics should be considered.

2. A – Elevation, rest and NSAIDs

Pain, erythema and a palpable cord-like structure around a cannula site strongly suggest a superficial thrombophlebitis. Management is by removing the cannula, along with elevation of the limb and NSAIDs for the pain. If there are any features to suggest infection then antibiotics should be commenced. Due to the risk of developing thrombophlebitis, peripheral cannulae should be replaced every 72 hours.

3. E – Reassurance and observation

Varicose veins are dilated, tortuous superficial veins. Most are idiopathic and are twice as common in females. Causes of secondary varicosities include previous DVT, arteriovenous fistulas, and inferior vena caval compression by pelvic malignancy or pregnancy.

Asymptomatic, uncomplicated varicose veins are best managed by reassurance and observation. Graded compression stockings can be used for small varicosities or in patients who are unfit for surgery, although many people find these uncomfortable. Intervention can be suggested if the patient finds the varicosities cosmetically unacceptable.

4. F – Saphenofemoral ligation

This woman has large varicosities in the distribution of the long saphenous vein. The long saphenous vein drains the medial side of the lower limb and runs from the dorsum of the foot to the saphenofemoral junction in the groin. The short saphenous vein drains the lateral aspect of the limb and empties into the popliteal vein behind the knee. Surgery for varicosities is indicated in grossly dilated or symptomatic varices, in patients with venous skin changes and in those who suffer haemorrhage from a varicosity. Varicose veins in the distribution of the long saphenous vein are treated with saphenofemoral ligation, where the long saphenous vein is stripped to the knee and all its branches ligated. Short saphenous varicosities are treated with saphenopopliteal ligation. Smaller varicose venules can be managed surgically using stab avulsions, where 2–3 mm incisions are made and the veins are pulled out using hooks. Surgery for varicose veins only works if the deep venous system is intact.

Saphenous, from Greek *saphenes* = obviously visible.

Sclerotherapy involves the injection of a sclerosant (e.g. phenol) into the vein in order to obliterate the lumen. It is useful for small, superficial varicosities found below the knee. Patients are required to wear compression stockings for 2 weeks following sclerotherapy.

5. H – Split-skin grafting

This woman has a venous ulcer. Venous ulceration is usually due to incompetence of the deep leg veins (deep venous insufficiency) and is most common in older females. Deep venous insufficiency can be accompanied by progressive skin changes, including oedema, pigmentation (haemosiderin deposition), eczema and lipodermatosclerosis (where the subcutaneous tissues are replaced by thick fibrous tissue). The final skin change is ulceration, which usually occurs around the medial malleolus (the medial gaiter area).

Venous ulcers are shallow and flat and only mildly painful. Arterial ulceration is often deep and painful. Before treating venous ulcers, it is important to exclude an arterial component to the ulceration. The ankle–brachial pressure index (ABPI) is calculated by dividing the systolic blood pressure in the ankle by the higher of the two systolic pressures in the arms. An ABPI of 1.0 is considered normal (i.e. the ankle and arm systolic pressure should be similar). An ABPI <0.8 (i.e. the ankle pressure is lower than the arm's) suggests peripheral arterial disease. The first-line management for venous ulceration is compression bandaging with prior excision of necrotic tissue. However, compression cannot be applied to someone with arterial disease, as this will further exacerbate symptoms. For this reason, anyone with suspected venous ulceration should have an ABPI measurement to help exclude arterial disease before compression bandaging is applied. If the ABPI is <0.8 then the arterial component of ulceration should be addressed first.

This woman has an ABPI of 0.9 and hence was treated with compression bandaging. This has failed, and split-skin grafting is the next management

step. Split-skin grafting is indicated in people with venous ulceration that has failed to improve after 12 weeks of compression bandaging or is >10 cm^2. Split-skin grafts involve removing a partial-thickness layer of skin (containing the epidermis and a part of the dermis) from another part of the patient's body and grafting it to the ulcerated area.

Practice Paper 2: Questions

THEME 1: HAEMATURIA

Options

A. Acute cystitis
B. Benign prostatic hyperplasia
C. Bladder calculi
D. Glomerulonephritis
E. Nephroblastoma
F. Polycystic kidney disease
G. Pyelonephritis
H. Renal cell carcinoma
I. Renal tract calculi
J. Transitional cell carcinoma of the bladder
K. Squamous cell carcinoma of the bladder

For each of the following people presenting with haematuria, select the most appropriate diagnosis. Each option may be used once, more than once or not at all.

1. A 34-year-old man presents with painless frank haematuria. He has a history of back pain and mentions that he had a sister who died earlier in the year from a bleed in her brain. He is a non-smoker. On examination, his blood pressure is 170/110 mmHg and both kidneys are palpable.
2. A 58-year-old man presents with painless frank haematuria. He has attended his general practitioner several times in the previous months for recurrent urinary tract infections. He is a smoker with a 100 pack-year history.
3. A 48-year-old woman presents to the emergency department with sudden-onset loin pain that radiates to her groin and haematuria. She has no significant past medical history. On examination, her temperature is 36.7°C and there is no abnormality.
4. A 58-year-old man presents with pain on passing urine and haematuria. He also admits to frequency of urination. The pain is experienced in the suprapubic region and is worse at the end of micturition. Abdominal examination reveals no abnormality.

5. A 48-year-old man presents with haematuria. He feels under the weather and has lost a stone in weight over the past month. On examination, he has left-sided lumbar pain and a left-sided varicocele. His kidney is palpable on the left side. A per rectum exam demonstrates no abnormality.

THEME 2: ARTERIAL BLOOD GASES

Options

A. Fully compensated metabolic acidosis
B. Fully compensated metabolic alkalosis
C. Fully compensated respiratory acidosis
D. Fully compensated respiratory alkalosis
E. Metabolic acidosis (not compensated)
F. Metabolic alkalosis (not compensated)
G. Respiratory acidosis (not compensated)
H. Respiratory alkalosis (not compensated)
I. Type I respiratory failure
J. Type II respiratory failure

For each of the following presentations, select the most appropriate acid–base abnormality. Each option may be used once, more than once or not at all.

Reference ranges: pO_2 > 11.0 kPa, pCO_2 4.6–6.0 kPa, bicarbonate 22–28 mmol/L, pH 7.35–7.45.

1. A 38-year-old man presents with severe epigastric pain and vomiting. His arterial blood gases are pH 7.48, pO_2 12.7, pCO_2 5.0, bicarbonate 33.
2. An 18-year-old woman who has a history of polyuria and polydipsia presents with reduced consciousness and apparent shortness of breath. Her blood gases show pH 7.29, pO_2 15.2, pCO_2 2.6, bicarbonate 16.
3. A 59-year-old man is admitted with chest pain and a purulent cough. His arterial blood gases are pH 7.32, pO_2 12.0, pCO_2 7.2, bicarbonate 26.
4. A 70-year-old man is returned to the ward following a transurethral resection of the prostate. You are called to see him because he is confused. Blood gases show pH 7.36, pO_2 7.0, pCO_2 5.0, bicarbonate 26.
5. A 22-year-old woman is admitted following a multiple overdose. She appears to be breathing heavily, so a blood gas is taken. The results show pH 7.38, pO_2 12.0, pCO_2 3.8, bicarbonate 18.

THEME 3: LOWER LIMB NERVE LESIONS

Options

A. Common peroneal nerve
B. Femoral nerve
C. Lateral femoral cutaneous nerve
D. Lateral plantar nerve
E. Medial plantar nerve
F. Obturator nerve

G. Sciatic nerve
H. Saphenous nerve
I. Sural nerve
J. Tibial nerve

For each of the following people presenting with neurological problems, select the most likely nerve involved. Each option may be used once, more than once or not at all.

1. A 42-year-old woman presents to the general practitioner complaining of intermittent pain in her right thigh. The pain is sharp and is relieved by sitting down. On examination, you note that she is obese. There is no deficit in tone or power in the lower limbs.
2. An 18-year-old man was previously admitted to the orthopaedic ward with an ankle fracture, which was managed with a plaster cast. After the cast is removed, the man is unable to dorsiflex his foot.
3. A 35-year-old man is taken to theatre after fracturing his hip in a motorcycle accident. During the postoperative period, it is noticed that he is unable to dorsiflex or plantarflex his foot. There is no sensation below the knee except in the medial aspect of the leg.
4. An 18-year-old woman is involved in a road traffic collision. Her left knee had hit the dashboard of the car. On arrival at the emergency department, she is unable to flex her toes on the left side. Examination reveals an absence of the ankle jerk and loss of sensation over the sole of the foot.
5. A 27-year-old man is stabbed in the groin during a bar fight. He attends the emergency department as he is unable to extend his knee. On examination, the knee jerk is absent and there is loss of sensation over the anterior thigh and medial aspect of the leg.

THEME 4: INVESTIGATION OF GASTROINTESTINAL BLEEDING

Options

A. Adrenaline injection
B. Angiography
C. Barium meal
D. Colonoscopy
E. Oesophagogastroduodenoscopy
F. Proctosigmoidoscopy
G. Sclerotherapy
H. Urgent laparotomy

For each of the following people presenting with gastrointestinal bleeding, select the next appropriate investigation. Each option may be used once, more than once or not at all.

1. A 76-year-old woman is admitted to the emergency department with a history of abdominal pain, passing blood per rectum and haematemesis.

An urgent upper and lower gastrointestinal colonoscopy are performed, but no active bleeding can be noted. The patient is showing signs of hypovolaemic shock and is still passing melaena. Her haemoglobin drops by 4 g/dL over the space of 4 hours.

2. A 63-year-old woman presents with haematemesis. After initial management, she is sent for an upper gastrointestinal endoscopy. The endoscopist sees a bleeding gastric ulcer with a vessel at the base.
3. A 67-year-old woman presents with fresh rectal bleeding. She also admits to a history of left-sided abdominal pain that is relieved by passing stools. Examination is unremarkable and the patient is haemodynamically stable.
4. A 42-year-old man presents with fresh blood loss per rectum. There is no haematemesis or melaena. He has no history of similar problems. On examination, his pulse is 138 and blood pressure 80/42.
5. A 45-year-old woman presents with a 4-week history of passing blood per rectum. She complains of seeing small amounts of bright red blood on the toilet paper and in the pan. The patient is otherwise well.

THEME 5: DIAGNOSIS OF BREAST DISEASE

Options

A. Breast abscess
B. Breast cancer
C. Breast cyst
D. Fat necrosis
E. Fibroadenoma
F. Galactocele
G. Galactorrhoea
H. Gynaecomastia
I. Lactating breast
J. Mondor disease
K. Paget disease
L. Peau d'orange
M. Simple obesity

For each of the following people presenting with breast disease, select the most likely diagnosis. Each option may be used once, more than once or not at all.

1. A 43-year-old woman attends the breast clinic complaining of a sudden pain and swelling in her right breast. On examination, a single, fluctuant swelling is palpable. Fine-needle aspiration reveals clear fluid.
2. A 24-year-old woman presents 5 weeks after the birth of her second child with a painful left breast. On examination, there is a 4 cm area of inflammation and erythema lateral to the nipple, with an associated underlying lump.

3. A 52-year-old obese woman comes to the breast clinic with an irregular 2 cm firm lump in her left breast. On questioning, she admits to recent trauma of the area. Core biopsy of the lesion is reported as B2.
4. A 24-year-old man complains of a soft swelling around his left nipple that has increased in size over the last year. He has no significant past medical history but admits to being a frequent user of cannabis. His body mass index is 21. On examination, there is no discharge, skin changes or axillary lymphadenopathy.
5. A 54-year-old woman presents with a 1-week history of pain in her left breast. On examination, you feel an indurated, tender, cord-like structure running down the anterior surface of the breast.

THEME 6: LOCAL ANAESTHETIC AGENTS

Options

A. Bupivicaine alone
B. Bupivicaine with adrenaline
C. Cocaine
D. Lidocaine alone
E. Lidocaine with adrenaline
F. Lidocaine/prilocaine mixture
G. Prilocaine

For each of the following scenarios, select the most appropriate local anaesthetic. Each option may be used once, more than once or not at all.

1. A 3-year-old boy presents with diarrhoea and vomiting. On examination, he is clinically dehydrated, so you decide that he needs intravenous fluids.
2. An 18-year-old woman presents with a laceration to her left middle finger that requires suturing.
3. A 65-year-old woman attends the emergency department with a Colles fracture following a fall. She requires anaesthesia before manipulation of the affected wrist.
4. A 58-year-old man is having a spinal anaesthetic before a hip replacement.
5. A 67-year-old needs a catheter insertion to manage acute urinary retention.

THEME 7: DIAGNOSIS OF JAUNDICE

Options

A. Alcoholic liver disease
B. Ascending cholangitis
C. Carcinoma of the head of the pancreas
D. Choledocholithiasis
E. Crigler–Najjar syndrome
F. Duodenal carcinoma

G. Gilbert syndrome
H. Hepatocellular carcinoma
I. Primary biliary cirrhosis

For each of the following people presenting with jaundice, select the most likely diagnosis. Each option may be used once, more than once or not at all.

1. A 25-year-old woman presents with a 2-week history of vague abdominal pain and worsening jaundice. She also complains of passing pale motions. The patient underwent a total colectomy for familial adenomatous polyposis at the age of 20. There is no abnormality on abdominal examination.
2. A 44-year-old woman presents with a 1-month history of jaundice associated with fatigue, itching and dark urine. She has a history of early-onset rheumatoid arthritis. On examination, she appears very jaundiced and has multiple xanthelasmas around her eyes. Abdominal examination is unremarkable.
3. A 65-year-old man presents with a 1-month history of worsening jaundice and itching. He has lost 2 stone in weight over this time but denies experiencing any pain. On examination, the abdomen is soft and a mass is palpable in the right upper quadrant.
4. A 28-year-old man attends the emergency department with a productive cough and malaise. His routine bloods on admission show a bilirubin level of 45 μmol/L. The remainder of his liver function tests are normal.
5. A 48-year-old man is brought to hospital by his wife as he has developed jaundice over the last few days. He is slightly confused and is unable to give a clear history. On examination, he has a distended, tense abdomen and dilated superficial veins around his umbilicus. His liver is not palpable.

THEME 8: THYROID DISEASE

Options

A. Anaplastic carcinoma
B. de Quervain thyroiditis
C. Follicular carcinoma
D. Graves disease
E. Hashimoto thyroiditis
F. Haemorrhage into a cyst
G. Medullary carcinoma
H. Papillary carcinoma
I. Riedel thyroiditis
J. Struma ovarii
K. Toxic multinodular goitre

For each of the following people presenting with neck lumps, select the most likely diagnosis. Each option may be used once, more than once or not at all.

1. A 25-year-old woman presents to the clinic with a slowly enlarging lump on the left side of her neck. She denies any other symptoms. On examination, there is a 2 cm smooth, regular, firm lump associated that moves up with swallowing but not with tongue protrusion. Lymph nodes are palpable in the left side of the neck.
2. A 54-year-old man presents to clinic with a midline neck mass that has been increasing in size over a few months. On examination, the thyroid gland is enlarged, firm and irregular, although the patient does not complain of any pain. No cervical nodes are palpable. A core biopsy is taken and the histology report denies the presence of malignancy.
3. A 42-year-old woman presents to the general practitioner with a large goitre, which she admits to having for a long time. More recently, she has been suffering with constipation, lethargy and weight gain. On examination, her pulse is 64/min and regular. She has a diffusely enlarged, smooth, firm goitre. No lymph nodes are palpable.
4. A 46-year-old woman presents to the emergency department with palpitations. She is clearly nervous and describes having multiple paroxysms of fast palpitations over the preceding fortnight. On examination, you find an enlarged, lumpy thyroid gland that is not fixed to the overlying skin.
5. An 84-year-old woman presents with a lump in her neck that was first noticed last month and has since been growing rapidly. On further questioning, she admits to problems swallowing her food. On examination, there is a 5 cm irregular, hard mass on the left side that is fixed to the overlying skin.

THEME 9: MANAGEMENT OF SKIN CONDITIONS

Options

A. 5-Fluorouracil
B. Analgesia
C. Cryotherapy
D. Fluid resuscitation
E. Intravenous antibiotics
F. Oral antibiotics
G. Surgical debridement and intravenous antibiotics
H. Surgical excision
I. Reassurance

For each of the following presentations, select the most appropriate management plan. Each option may be used once, more than once or not at all.

1. A 7-year-old boy is brought to the general practitioner by his father because he has longstanding freckling in his mouth. On examination, the child has multiple bluish-black macular lesions around his lips and nose. He is otherwise well.
2. A 3-year-old girl is brought to the emergency department by her mother with multiple yellow crusty blistering lesions on her face and arms. The lesions are itchy and occasionally bleed. The girl's older brother is suffering similar complaints.
3. A 67-year-old woman presents with a temperature and feeling unwell. She has a large area of erythema and swelling on her right leg, which is becoming necrotic. This started when she hit her leg on a stool a few days ago, but since then the erythema and necrosis has spread rapidly.
4. A 22-year-old man presents to his general practitioner with a lesion on the back of his neck. On examination, the lesion is 1 cm in size, painless and mobile. It is attached to the overlying skin but not to the underlying muscle and it has a central punctum. There is no palpable cervical lymphadenopathy. The man is worried about the cosmetic appearance.
5. A 34-year-old man presents to the emergency department with redness and swelling of his right cheek. On examination, the area of erythema is well demarcated and is hot to touch. His temperature is 38.1°C and he feels unwell.

THEME 10: NECK LUMPS

Options

A. Branchial cyst
B. Cervical rib
C. Chemodectoma
D. Dermoid cyst
E. Pleomorphic adenoma
F. Salivary duct carcinoma
G. Salivary gland stone
H. Sternocleidomastoid tumour
I. Thyroglossal cyst
J. Virchow node

For each of the following people with neck lumps, select the most likely diagnosis. Each option may be used once, more than once or not at all.

1. A 27-year-old woman presents with pain and paraesthesia in her left arm. On examination, you note problems specifically in the medial aspect of the arm. There is also a firm lump palpable in her neck on the left side.
2. A 48-year-old woman presents with a lump in her neck, which has been slowly growing over the past 6 months. On examination, there is a firm, mobile, hard, painless lump in the left neck near the angle of the jaw. There is no transmitted pulsation. The woman has not lost use of her facial muscles.

3. A 35-year-old man presents with a slowly enlarging neck mass. On examination, the mass is painless and mobilizes side-to-side only. Pressing on the mass demonstrates a pulsation and makes the patient feel faint.
4. A 2-month-old boy is taken to his general practitioner with a lump in the left side of his neck. On examination, the baby has his head tilted towards the side of the lump, which itself is firm and appears to be attached to the underlying muscle.
5. A 57-year-old man presents with a lump in his neck, which has been present since he had a rose-thorn prick him in the area when he was gardening. He is otherwise well. On examination, there is a 1 cm mobile, painless lump just under his left earlobe.

THEME 11: PAEDIATRIC ORTHOPAEDIC CONDITIONS

Options

A. Developmental dysplasia of the hip
B. Genu varus
C. Osgood–Schlatter disease
D. Perthes disease
E. Septic arthritis
F. Slipped upper femoral epiphysis
G. Spontaneous haemarthrosis
H. Talipes equinovarus
I. Transient synovitis
J. Still's disease

For each of the following presentations, select the most likely diagnosis. Each option may be used once, more than once or not at all.

1. A 6-week-old baby boy is visited by the community midwife for a routine neonatal check. She notices that his feet are abnormally inverted. There is no other joint abnormality in the legs.
2. A 12-year-old boy fell off his bike and hurt his left knee. The knee promptly swelled to twice its size and was tender. His father explains that this has happened on several previous occasions and that his brother-in-law suffers similar problems.
3. A 15-year-old girl presents with difficulty walking on her left leg because of pain. On examination, she is pyrexial and her left ankle is hot, swollen and tender.
4. A 4-year-old boy is brought to the general practitioner by his parents because they are worried about the way he stands. On examination, the boy stands with his legs bowed. There is no swelling or tenderness in the joints of the lower limbs.
5. A 14-year-old boy presents with pain in his right knee that is worse when he plays football. On examination, he is apyrexial but the left tibial tubercle is enlarged and painful.

THEME 12: GASTROINTESTINAL POLYPS

Options

A. Adenomatous polyp
B. Hamartomatous polyp
C. Juvenile polyp
D. Metaplastic polyp
E. Pseudopolyp
F. Villous adenoma

For each of the following scenarios, select the most likely diagnosis. Each option may be used once, more than once or not at all.

1. A 16-year-old girl requests a colonoscopy after her older brother had recently been diagnosed with colon cancer aged 21. Her mother died at the age of 28 from a caecal tumour. The colonoscopy shows multiple polyps throughout the colon. Histology shows these to be benign.
2. A 45-year-old man undergoes an upper gastrointestinal endoscopy following an episode of haematemesis. He is found to have multiple polyps in his duodenum, which are later found to be benign. It is noticed that he has multiple freckles around his lips.
3. A 40-year-old man presents with a 2-week history of diarrhoea and muscle weakness. A colonoscopy shows a 2 cm sessile growth that has multiple projections.
4. A 36-year-old man with known ulcerative colitis undergoes a routine colonoscopy. A number of small projections can be seen throughout the bowel. These are confirmed as benign.
5. A 12-year-old girl presents with one episode of per rectum bleeding. A lower gastrointestinal endoscopy detects the presence of a single, large lesion that appears to be on a 'stalk'.

THEME 13: FEMORAL NECK FRACTURES

Options

A. Analgesia alone
B. Cannulated screws
C. Dynamic hip screws
D. Hemiarthroplasty
E. Plaster cast
F. Total hip replacement

For each of the following femoral neck fractures, select the most appropriate management. Each option may be used once, more than once or not at all.

1. A 50-year-old man presents with hip pain after falling over at work. He was previously fit and well. An X-ray shows a minimally displaced intracapsular fracture of the right femoral neck.

2. A 68-year-old woman presents with an inter-trochanteric fracture following a fall. She has no significant comorbidities.
3. A 72-year-old woman presents with an undisplaced femoral neck fracture. She has hypertension but no other significant past medical history.
4. A 85-year-old woman fell while washing and sustained a displaced subcapital femoral neck fracture. She has a history of ischaemic heart disease, hypertension and diabetes.
5. A 68-year-old man who has osteoarthritis of his right hip is admitted to hospital after a fall. He is found to have a displaced intracapsular fracture of the right femoral neck.

THEME 14: DIAGNOSIS OF GROIN LUMPS

Options

A. Epididymo-orchitis
B. False femoral aneurysm
C. Hydrocele
D. Mumps orchitis
E. Reducible indirect inguinal hernia
F. Saphena varix
G. Sebaceous cyst
H. Strangulated femoral hernia
I. Strangulated inguinal hernia
J. Testicular torsion
K. Testicular tumour
L. Varicocele

For each of the following people presenting with groin lumps, select the most appropriate diagnosis. Each option may be used once, more than once or not at all.

1. A 28-year-old man presents with a large left-sided scrotal swelling that is causing slight discomfort. On examination, the swelling is soft but does not transilluminate. You cannot get above it and it disappears on lying flat, but there is no cough impulse.
2. A 24-year-old man presents with a swelling in his right scrotum that has been increasing in size over the last year. On examination, the swelling is non-tender and fluctuant and it transilluminates. It is possible to get above the swelling, but the testis is not palpable.
3. A 64-year-old man presents with a small lump on the skin of his left scrotum. On examination, the lump is tethered to the skin but not attached to any underlying structure, and it is not tender.
4. A 7-year-old boy who has been admitted to hospital with viral meningitis acutely develops a painful swelling in his testicle. On examination, the boy is pyrexial and the swelling is tender.

5. A 52-year-old woman presents with a swelling on her left thigh, below and lateral to the pubic tubercle. On examination, the swelling is bluish, non-tender, non-pulsatile and compressible. The patient is otherwise well.

THEME 15: CLASSIFICATION OF HERNIAS

Options

A. Incarcerated
B. Obstructed
C. Perforated
D. Reducible
E. Richter
F. Sliding
G. Strangulated

For each of the following scenarios, choose the most appropriate description for the hernia. Each option may be used once, more than once or not at all.

1. A 63-year-old man presents with a lump in his groin. On examination, there is a mass in the scrotum, which disappears on lying down. There is no pain or erythema associated with the lump and the patient is asymptomatic. When the patient coughs, an impulse can be felt over the hernia.
2. A 34-year-old man presents with a lump in the lower midline of his abdomen. On examination, you note that the lump is in the lower end of a midline laparotomy scar. The lump is 4 cm in size and the contents cannot be returned to the abdomen by pressure, and there is no cough impulse. The lump itself is neither painful nor erythematous.
3. A 48-year-old woman presents with a small lump in the groin, below and lateral to the pubic tubercle. She also complains of vomiting and colicky abdominal pain. On examination, the lump is 1 cm in diameter and is painful and erythematous. There is no cough impulse.
4. A 45-year-old man who has a known direct inguinal hernia presents to the emergency department as his hernia has become painful over the last few hours. On examination, the hernia is irreducible, tender and erythematous. The patient denies any colicky abdominal pain, vomiting or constipation.
5. A 78-year-old woman with a previous epigastric hernia presents with severe abdominal pain and vomiting. On examination, she is pyrexial and tachycardic and has a diffusely painful, rigid abdomen. No bowel sounds can be heard. Her hernia is noted to be erythematous and irreducible.

THEME 16: INVESTIGATION OF VASCULAR DISEASE

Options

A. Ankle–brachial pressure index
B. Contrast angiography

C. CT scan
D. Duplex Doppler ultrasound
E. Hand-held Doppler
F. Magnetic resonance venogram
G. No investigation required
H. Venography

For each of the following people presenting with vascular disease, select the next most appropriate investigation. Each option may be used once, more than once or not at all.

1. A 69-year-old woman presents with sudden-onset difficulty in walking and slurred speech. On examination, power was reduced on the right side in both upper and lower limbs. There was also weakness of the right side of the face, with forehead sparing. Her symptoms resolved soon after admission.
2. A 59-year-old man presents with a cramping pain in his left calf that occurs with walking. The pain usually occurs after walking 100 metres and is relieved by rest.
3. A 29-year-old woman presents with bilateral lower leg varicosities that are causing her embarrassment and discomfort, and for which she is requesting surgery. The surgeon in the clinic wants to elicit where the site of venous incompetence is.
4. A 68-year-old man presents with left lower limb claudication that prevents him from walking further than 100 metres. The ankle–brachial pressure index is 0.64.
5. A 68-year-old man presents with sudden-onset severe epigastric pain that radiates to his back. He has no past medical history. On examination, you find that he is cold and sweaty. His pulse is 116/min and his blood pressure is 80/45 mmHg.

Practice Paper 2: Answers

THEME 1: HAEMATURIA

1. F – Polycystic kidney disease

Polycystic kidney disease is an autosomal dominant condition caused by a defect in the PKD gene on chromosome 6. Cystic changes are bilateral and the kidneys gradually enlarge. Clinical features of polycystic kidney disease include bilateral upper quadrant masses (cystic enlargement of the kidneys), dull loin pain, frank haematuria (from rupture of a cyst into the renal pelvis), hypertension and eventually chronic renal failure (in 10% of cases). Patients may also experience urinary tract infections and renal colic symptoms. Around 20% of cases also develop a polycystic liver and there is an association between polycystic disease and berry aneurysms in the circle of Willis (which can result in subarachnoid haemorrhage). Cysts can also develop in the pancreas and spleen.

Thomas Willis, English anatomist and physician (1621–1675).

2. J – Transitional cell carcinoma of the bladder

The presentation of painless frank haematuria in a male smoker should alert you to transitional cell carcinoma (TCC) of the bladder. Another risk factor for developing TCC is working in the dye or rubber industries, due to the excretion of carcinogens such as beta-naphthylamine in the urine. Patients present with painless frank haematuria or with multiple urinary tract infections.

Squamous cell carcinoma of the bladder is much more common in developing countries and occurs as a complication of infection with *Schistosoma*, a flatworm parasite that lives in freshwater snails and can cause chronic inflammation in the human bladder. The worm is able to penetrate through exposed skin and lay eggs in the nervous system.

3. I – Renal tract calculi

Renal calculi are slightly more common in males and usually occur in middle age. Although some calculi are silent, many present with sudden-onset pain that radiates from the loin to the groin (ureteric colic). The pain results from the squeezing, stretching and spasm of the ureters. The condition is usually associated with microscopic haematuria, although visible haematuria may occasionally occur. There are five anatomical sites where a stone may impact: the ureteropelvic junction, where the iliac artery crosses the ureter, the juxtaposition with the vas deferens (males) or the broad ligament (females), where the ureter enters the bladder wall, and finally the ureteric orifice.

Risk factors for developing renal stones include urinary tract infections, urinary stasis (e.g. bladder outflow obstruction), chronic dehydration and hypercalcaemia. The most common type of renal stone is the calcium oxalate stone (60%), which is radio-opaque. Other renal stones include calcium phosphate calculi (33%), which tend to form in alkaline urine, especially in the presence of *Proteus* infection (radio-opaque). Phosphate calculi may enlarge to fill the whole renal collecting system (staghorn calculus). More rare renal calculi include urate stones (radiolucent) and cysteine stones (radio-opaque). A kidney-ureter-bladder (KUB) plain X-ray shows up around 90% of renal calculi, although some hospitals use spiral CT as the first-line investigation for renal stones.

4. C – Bladder calculi

Bladder calculi present with the triad of dysuria, haematuria and frequency. There may also be intermittent halting of urinary flow as the stone blocks the urethral meatus in the bladder. The pain is suprapubic and radiates to the perineum and tip of the penis. Pain and haematuria are worse at the end of micturition as the bladder contracts against the stone. Bladder calculi are of the same types as renal calculi (oxalate, phosphate, urate and cysteine). Bladder stones may originate in the kidney and travel to the bladder or may occur *de novo* in the bladder. Stones that arise in the bladder are due to stasis, infection or the presence of a long-term indwelling catheter.

5. H – Renal cell carcinoma

Renal cell adenocarcinoma (also known as hypernephroma or Grawitz tumour) is the most common renal tumour, occurring most often in males over the age of 40. It presents with a triad of haematuria (with the occasional clot), flank pain (in 40%) and a palpable abdominal mass (in 20%). A new left-sided varicocele may occur (in 1%) in men with renal tumours due to obstruction of the left testicular vein (the left testicular vein drains into the renal vein, whereas the right testicular vein drains directly into the inferior vena cava). Other features are hypertension (from hyperaldosteronism), polycythaemia (from excess erythropoietin production) and hypercalcaemia (from surplus hydroxylation of vitamin D). If obstruction of the inferior vena cava occurs, bilateral leg oedema can result. Renal cell carcinomas can be associated with congenital conditions such as von Hippel–Lindau (renal cell carcinoma + phaeochromocytoma + central nervous system haemangiomas) and tuberous sclerosis (multisystem tumours + developmental delay + seizures + characteristic skin lesions (adenoma sebaceum, shagreen patch, ash-leaf macules and subungual fibromas)). Renal cell carcinomas are golden-yellow in colour. Renal cell carcinoma has many histological subtypes of which clear cell carcinoma is the most common (60–70% of cases). Cure is achieved in up to half of all patients with early stage disease.

Tuberous sclerosis, from Latin *tuber* = swelling and Greek *skleros* = hard; describing the pathological finding of thick, firm gyri on postmortem examination of the brain.

Paul Albert Grawitz, German pathologist (1850–1932).
Eugen von Hippel, German ophthalmologist (1867–1939).
Arvid Vilhelm Lindau, Swedish pathologist (1892–1958).

THEME 2: ARTERIAL BLOOD GASES

Simple interpretation of arterial blood gases is usually all that is required in final EMQs. The pH value shows if the gas is acidotic (<7.35) or alkalotic (>7.45). Next, you need to find out if the alkalosis or acidosis is due to a metabolic or respiratory cause – this is done by looking at the pCO_2 and bicarbonate levels. There are two things you need to bear in mind before continuing: (1) carbon dioxide is acidic and bicarbonate is alkaline; and (2) bicarbonate equates to 'metabolic' and pCO_2 means 'respiratory'. An alkalosis can be due to either a high bicarbonate ('metabolic alkalosis') or a low pCO_2 ('respiratory alkalosis'). Conversely, an acidosis can be caused by either a low bicarbonate ('metabolic acidosis') or a high pCO_2 ('respiratory acidosis').

In some cases of blood gas disturbance, the body has time to compensate. In other words, whichever chemical is causing the imbalance is counteracted by the opposite one. For example, if there is a high bicarbonate (metabolic alkalosis) then the pCO_2 starts to increase to bring in some acidity and counteract the alkalosis. If compensation is successful, the pH will return to within the normal range (7.35–7.45), even if the bicarbonate and pCO_2 levels are abnormal. It is important to realize that the body can never overcompensate, i.e. if there is an initial acidosis, the body can never make that into an alkalosis, and the pH will always remain on the acidic side of normal (<7.40). Similarly, a compensated alkalosis will always have a pH >7.40, on the alkalotic side of normal.

Respiratory failure is defined as a pO_2 <8.0. Type I respiratory failure occurs when there is hypoxia in the presence of a low or normal pCO_2. Type II respiratory failure is hypoxia in the presence of a high pCO_2.

1. F – Metabolic alkalosis (not compensated)

This man has an abnormal pH of 7.48, which is alkalotic (>7.45). Because the bicarbonate is high, we know this is a metabolic alkalosis. The pCO_2 is within the normal range and he is not hypoxic, so overall he has a metabolic alkalosis with no effort at compensation. This blood gas is explained by his vomiting, with a consequent loss of gastric acid.

2. E – Metabolic acidosis (not compensated)

This patient's pH is acidotic (<7.29). The low pCO_2 contributes to alkalosis but the low bicarbonate would cause an acidosis. The acidosis must therefore be due to the bicarbonate, with the carbon dioxide making an attempt to compensate but not quite managing. This is therefore a partially compensated metabolic acidosis and, along with the patient's presentation, suggests diabetic ketoacidosis.

3. G – Respiratory acidosis (not compensated)

The pH is 7.32 (an acidosis). The bicarbonate is normal but the carbon dioxide is high, so it must be this that is contributing to the acid–base imbalance (respiratory acidosis). Since there is no effort at compensation by bicarbonate, this is an uncompensated respiratory acidosis and could be due to an underlying chest infection.

4. I – Type I respiratory failure

The pH, pCO_2 and bicarbonate levels are normal in this case, so there is no acid–base disorder. However this man has hypoxia (pO_2 < 8), which denotes respiratory failure. Because the pCO_2 is not high, this is a type I respiratory failure. Hypoxia is a common cause of confusion.

5. A – Fully compensated metabolic acidosis

This woman has a normal pH but abnormal carbon dioxide and bicarbonate levels. Therefore there definitely is an acid–base imbalance, but it has been fully compensated. Because the pH is on the acidic side of normal (<7.40), you can safely say that the original disturbance was an acidosis. The low bicarbonate would cause the acidosis and the low pCO_2 would result in the compensatory alkalosis. Overall, this picture is a fully compensated metabolic acidosis, which could be accounted for by salicylate poisoning.

THEME 3: LOWER LIMB NERVE LESIONS

1. C – Lateral femoral cutaneous nerve

The lateral femoral cutaneous nerve can become trapped beneath the inguinal ligament where it attaches to the anterior superior iliac spine. It tends to occur in obese people or pregnant women. Nerve entrapment causes pain or a burning sensation in the lateral thigh (known as meralgia paraesthetica) with no motor abnormality. Pain is often caused by long periods of standing.

Meralgia, from Greek *meros* = thigh + *algos* = pain.

2. A – Common peroneal nerve

The common peroneal nerve (or common fibular nerve) is a branch of the sciatic nerve which supplies the dorsiflexors and evertor muscles of the foot and sensation to the lateral lower leg and upper foot. The common peroneal nerve lies in close proximity to the fibula and may become trapped by below-knee plaster casts or damaged with fibular fractures.

Features of common peroneal nerve lesions include lack of dorsiflexion (with a resulting foot drop) and loss of sensation in the anterolateral lower leg and dorsum of the foot (except for the lateral aspect of the foot, which is supplied by the sural nerve). The inability to dorsiflex the foot will result in a 'high-stepping' gait to ensure that it is not scraped along the ground.

3. G – Sciatic nerve

The sciatic nerve can be damaged with fracture dislocations of the hip or by misplaced gluteal injections. (Intramuscular injections should therefore be sited in the upper outer aspect of the buttock to avoid the sciatic nerve, which runs beneath the lower inner quadrant of the buttock.) Sciatic nerve palsy results in paralysis of the hamstrings and all the muscles of the leg and foot. Sensation is lost below the knee except for the medial leg (supplied by the saphenous nerve, a branch of the femoral nerve) and the upper calf (supplied by the posterior femoral cutaneous nerve).

4. J – Tibial nerve

The tibial nerve is particularly vulnerable to damage during posterior dislocations of the knee. It can also be compressed in the posterior tarsal tunnel behind the medial malleolus. A branch of the sciatic nerve, the tibial nerve supplies the flexor compartment of the leg (calf muscles). It also gives rise to the medial and lateral plantar nerves, which supply the intrinsic muscles of the foot as well as plantar sensation. Tibial nerve palsy results in loss of toe flexion, ankle inversion and the ankle jerk. Sensation over the plantar surface of the foot is lost. Affected patients walk with a shuffling gait, as the take-off phase of walking is impaired. There is loss of the lateral longitudinal arch of the foot, and atrophy of the intrinsic foot muscles eventually results in a claw-foot.

5. B – Femoral nerve

The femoral nerve enters the thigh via the femoral triangle, where it lies lateral to the femoral artery. It can easily be damaged by penetrating wounds, hip dislocations or thigh haematomas. The femoral nerve supplies motor branches to the quadriceps and sensory branches to the anterior thigh and medial calf (via the saphenous nerve). Femoral nerve palsies result in a loss of knee extension and loss of sensation over the anterior thigh and medial leg.

The saphenous nerve can be damaged during long saphenous vein surgery, particularly when the vein is stripped below the knee, resulting in loss of sensation to the medial aspect of the calf. The obturator nerve can be damaged in obstetric procedures and pelvic disease. Features of an obturator nerve palsy include loss of hip adduction and loss of sensation to the upper inner thigh. The sural nerve is a cutaneous sensory branch of the tibial nerve, which can be damaged during short saphenous vein surgery.

Lesions of the sural nerve result in a loss of sensation to the lateral side of the foot and little toe. Superior gluteal nerve lesions result in loss of hip abduction and a pelvic dip on walking (Trendelenburg gait). Inferior gluteal nerve lesions lead to loss of hip extension and buttock wasting.

THEME 4: INVESTIGATION OF GASTROINTESTINAL BLEEDING

1. B – Angiography

This woman is presenting with continuing melaena and hypovolaemic shock. There is therefore a bleed somewhere along the gastrointestinal tract. If both upper and lower endoscopies are negative, a mesenteric angiography will need to be performed to help source the site of the bleed. Large bleeds can be identified and the bleeding vessel embolised.

2. A – Adrenaline injection

If a bleeding ulcer is seen at endoscopy, the first step in management is injection of the ulcer with 1:10 000 adrenaline to achieve haemostasis.

3. D – Colonoscopy

The history is suggestive of diverticular disease. As the nature of the bleeding is most likely to be of lower gastrointestinal origin, a colonoscopy would be the most sensible first-line investigation. The bright red nature of the bleed is suggestive of bleeding from the left side of the colon. However, brisk bleeds from the ascending colon may also be bright red, so colonoscopy (rather than a sigmoidoscopy) is the investigation of choice here.

4. E – Oesophagogastroduodenoscopy

This patient is also presenting with fresh blood per rectum. However, unlike the woman in the previous scenario, there is nothing to suggest a lower GI cause and this patient is haemodynamically compromised. In this case, therefore, the first investigation to perform would be an oesophagogastroduodenoscopy (OGD) in order to rule out a bleeding peptic ulcer. An OGD can be both diagnostic and therapeutic.

5. F – Proctosigmoidoscopy

This woman is presenting with features of haemorrhoids. The first investigation to perform would be a proctosigmoidoscopy, which would confirm the presence of piles within the anus. This investigation is relatively simple and can be performed in outpatients. If no cause of this woman's bleeding could be found, a flexible sigmoidoscopy would be the next investigation.

THEME 5: DIAGNOSIS OF BREAST DISEASE

1. C – Breast cyst

Breast cysts typically present as a sudden, painful swelling in the breast. They are most common in the 40s. Diagnosis and treatment is by aspiration, which reveals a clear fluid. In 30% of cases, breast cysts recur – these require surgical excision. Occasionally, breast cyst aspirate is blood-stained, and this is suggestive of malignancy within the wall of the cyst. If this is the case, local excision of the lesion is required.

2. A – Breast abscess

Bacterial mastitis describes infection of a lactiferous duct by *Staphylococcus aureus,* which is transmitted by an infant's nasopharynx during lactation. It presents with cellulitis around the infected area, with pyrexia, tachycardia and a leukocytosis. A complication of bacterial mastitis is the formation of a breast abscess, resulting in a palpable lump (as has occurred in this case). The mainstay of treatment of bacterial mastitis is antibiotics. However if an abscess is present, it must be aspirated.

3. D – Fat necrosis

Fat necrosis is most common in obese, middle-aged women with a history of trauma to the area. It presents with a painless, irregular, firm lump in the breast and may be associated with skin thickening or retraction. The size of the lump usually decreases with time, but residual fat cysts may be left within the breast. The diagnosis of fat necrosis must be confirmed by core biopsy, as the presenting features may be similar to those of carcinoma.

Core biopsy results are signified using the following scale:

B1 normal
B2 benign breast tissue (as in this question)
B3 equivocal, probably benign
B4 suspicious, probably malignant
B5 malignant breast tissue

4. H – Gynaecomastia

Gynaecomastia is the benign proliferation of male breast tissue due to an imbalance of oestrogens and androgens. It is physiological (normal) in neonates, puberty and the elderly. There are many other causes of gynaecomastia; these include drugs (cimetidine, spironolactone, cannabis, oestrogen and steroids), renal failure, cirrhosis and testicular tumours. Obesity is not a cause of true gynaecomastia. Although most cases of gynaecomastia resolve spontaneously, excision can be offered if lesions do not settle or are symptomatic or embarrassing.

Gynaecomastia, from Latin *gynae* = woman + *mastia* = breast.

5. J – Mondor disease

Mondor disease is a rare condition describing thrombophlebitis of the superficial veins of the breast and anterior chest wall. It is characterized by a painful, inflamed subcutaneous cord that is tethered to the skin. When the arm on the affected side is raised, a shallow groove becomes apparent alongside the cord. Treatment is with rest and analgesia.

Henri Mondor, French surgeon (1885–1962).

THEME 6: LOCAL ANAESTHETIC AGENTS

Local anaesthetics are drugs that reversibly inhibit the propagation of nerve impulses. They work by transiently altering the neuronal membrane permeability to sodium ions.

1. F – Lidocaine/prilocaine mixture

Lidocaine/prilocaine mixture can be given as a topical emulsion preparation to children before inserting a cannula or taking bloods. It is marketed under the trade name Emla ('eutectic mixture of local anaesthetic') and the emulsion is left on for 30–60 minutes to allow full dermal anaesthesia to take place. A 'eutetic' mixture is one that contains equal amounts of each ingredient. For example, Emla contains 2.5% each of lidocaine and prilocaine. Other examples of topical local anaesthetics include Instillagel (lidocaine) used for urethral catheterization, and Xylocaine (lidocaine) spray given before upper gastrointestinal endoscopies. Amethocaine eye drops are used for conjunctival anaesthesia. Amethocaine is also available as a cream, and its onset of action of dermal anaesthesia is more rapid than that of Emla.

2. D – Lidocaine alone

Before suturing a finger, anaesthesia is produced by doing a ring block. This involves injection of 1–2 mL of local anaesthetic either side of the proximal phalanx at the level of the web space where the digital nerves run, producing anaesthesia along the entire length of the digit. Lidocaine is a quick-acting local anaesthetic and is appropriate for ring blocks. Adrenaline causes vasoconstriction and has the advantages of slowing systemic absorption and prolonging duration of action of local anaesthetics. However, local anaesthetics containing adrenaline must NEVER be used near end-arteries (e.g. digits and penis), as there is a risk of ischaemic necrosis. The maximum dose of plain lidocaine is 3 mg/kg and 7 mg/kg when combined with adrenaline.

3. G – Prilocaine

Before manipulation of Colles fractures, regional anaesthesia of the upper limb is required. This technique is known as a Bier block. A Bier block is performed by first squeezing the blood out of the limb, then inflating a tourniquet around the upper arm and injecting intravenous prilocaine into the arm distal to the tourniquet. The tourniquet prevents local anaesthetic from leaving the arm and blood from entering. Prilocaine is the best local anaesthetic to use for this procedure as it is the least cardiotoxic. The maximum dose of prilocaine is 6 mg/kg (or 9 mg/kg when combined with adrenaline).

August Bier, German surgeon (1861–1949).

4. A – Bupivicaine alone

Bupivicaine is a longer-acting anaesthetic that can be used without adrenaline for spinal or epidural anaesthesia. Bupivicaine can also be injected into surgical wounds with adrenaline to reduce postoperative pain for up to 20 hours. A mixture of bupivicaine and lidocaine is used for carpal tunnel surgery as it allows rapid onset of anaesthesia and longer-acting postoperative analgesia. Bupivicaine is contraindicated for intravenous regional anaesthesia (such as Bier block) as it is cardiotoxic. It has a maximum dose of 2 mg/kg when used alone and 3 mg/kg when combined with adrenaline.

5. D – Lidocaine alone

Lidocaine gel (Instillagel) is used before urethral catheter insertion to create anaesthesia of the area. See Part 1 for other uses of topical local anaesthesia.

Cocaine was the first compound to be used as a local anaesthetic. Its anaesthetic properties were discovered accidentally by Sigmund Freud (Austrian neurologist, psychiatrist and frequent cocaine user). Cocaine has since been used in ophthalmic and nasal operations. Side effects of cocaine include intense vasoconstriction and cardiotoxicity, so it has now largely been replaced by benzocaine and proparacaine for ENT use.

THEME 7: DIAGNOSIS OF JAUNDICE

1. F – Duodenal carcinoma

This woman has familial adenomatous polyposis (FAP), for which she underwent prophylactic colectomy. FAP is associated with the development of duodenal carcinoma, which tends to occur near the sphincter of Oddi. Such a tumour would result in the symptoms described in this scenario, namely abdominal pain and obstructive jaundice. FAP, like HNPCC (hereditary non-polyposis colorectal cancer), is an autosomal dominant genetic condition. Gardener syndrome is the combination of polyposis, osteomas, fibromas and sebaceous cysts.

2. I – Primary biliary cirrhosis

This woman has features of obstructive jaundice with xanthelasma and a history of autoimmune disease. The most likely diagnosis is primary biliary cirrhosis. Primary biliary cirrhosis (PBC) is an autoimmune condition that affects middle-aged women and is characterized by chronic inflammation and fibrosis of the interlobular bile ducts. Patients present with pruritus (the most common symptom), jaundice, xanthelasma and arthralgia. Some patients display features of portal hypertension, because PBC can result in cirrhosis. The majority of patients are positive for anti-mitochondrial antibody, but a liver biopsy is the diagnostic test. Symptomatic management of pruritus is with ursodeoxycholic acid, cholestyramine and antihistamines. The disease will progress unless a liver transplant is offered.

Xanthelasma, from Greek *xanthos* = yellow + *elasma* = plate.

3. C – Carcinoma of the head of the pancreas

This older man has painless progressive jaundice and weight loss with a palpable gallbladder – features that point strongly to carcinoma of the head of the pancreas. Pancreatic carcinoma is the fifth most common cancer in the West, occurring most often in the over-60 age group. Sixty percent of tumours are located in the head of the pancreas, and these often obstruct the outflow of bile in the common bile duct. Risk factors for pancreatic carcinoma include diabetes, smoking and excess alcohol consumption. The classic presentation of carcinoma of the pancreas is with painless progressive jaundice. However, some patients complain of a dull epigastric pain that radiates to the back. If the tumour obstructs the common bile duct, there is obstruction of bile flow, resulting in a full, palpable gallbladder. Remember Courvoisier's law: 'If in the presence of jaundice the gallbladder is palpable then the cause is unlikely to be stones' (i.e. it is likely to be a tumour!). Suspected pancreatic tumours should be delineated with a CT scan. Operative excision of pancreatic carcinomas is by Whipple's procedure. In this procedure, four things are removed: the pancreatic head, which contains the tumours; the common bile duct and gallbladder; the distal stomach; and some of the duodenum. Three anastomoses must be created: a hepato-jejenostomy, a pancreatic jejunostomy, and finally a gastro-jejenostomy. The risk of having a major complication from the procedure is approximately 1 in 3. Of these anastomoses, the pancreatic jejunostomy is the one that has the highest risk of leaking due to the proteolytic nature of the pancreatic secretions. Overall, inoperable pancreatic tumours have a very poor prognosis – most people are dead within 6 months.

Thrombophlebitis migrans is characterized by the formation of recurrent clots in superficial veins in different areas of the body. It is a skin condition that is strongly associated with pancreatic carcinoma, occurring due to the hypercoagulable state associated with malignancy. The association of thrombophlebitis migrans with pancreatic carcinoma is known as Trousseau's sign, named after the doctor who first described it (and who incidentally died of pancreatic cancer himself).

Ludwig Georg Courvoisier, Swiss surgeon (1843–1918).

Armand Trousseau, French physician (1801–1867).

4. G – Gilbert syndrome

Gilbert syndrome is an autosomal dominant partial deficiency in glucuronosyltransferase, the enzyme that is required to conjugate bilirubin. People with this condition have a mildly raised non-haemolytic isolated unconjugated hyperbilirubinaemia, especially when they are acutely unwell. The remainder of the liver function tests are unaffected. Diagnosis of Gilbert syndrome can be made following a thorough history and examination to exclude an alternative cause for hyperbilirubinaemia and a full blood count should be checked for the presence of reticulocytes and anaemia. Another congenital cause of hyperbilirubinaemia is Crigler–Najjar syndrome, an autosomal recessive total deficiency in glucuronosyltransferase resulting in unconjugated jaundice. This condition causes severe brain damage in the early years of life. Dubin–Johnson and Rotor syndromes both result in impaired excretion of bile with a consequent conjugated hyperbilirubinaemia.

Nicholas Augustin Gilbert, French physician (1858–1927).

5. A – Alcoholic liver disease

Alcoholic liver disease (ALD) can present with jaundice, abdominal pain, malnutrition, ascites and encephalopathy. Other signs of ALD include palmar erythema, spider naevi, purpura, hair loss, gynaecomastia and testicular atrophy. The presence of dilated superficial veins around the umbilicus occurs secondary to portal hypertension and is called caput medusae. In susceptible people, excess alcohol ingestion eventually causes liver cirrhosis. Although ALD is potentially reversible, once cirrhosis occurs, a liver transplant is required.

Caput medusae, from Latin 'head of Medusa', a character from Greek mythology who had snakes for hair and turned people to stone if they looked her in the eye.

Cirrhosis, from Greek *kirrhos* = orangey-brown; describing the appearance of the cirrhosed liver.

THEME 8: THYROID DISEASE

1. H – Papillary carcinoma

The majority (70%) of thyroid tumours are papillary adenocarcinomas. Twenty percent are follicular carcinomas. Both of these tumours occur most commonly in adolescents and young adults, who present with a discrete thyroid nodule. Papillary tumours may be multifocal and they spread to lymph nodes (as in this case). Histological analysis demonstrates a characteristic 'Orphan Annie eye' appearance of the nuclei (they appear empty). It has 5-year survival of 90%.

Follicular tumours occur as a single encapsulated lesion, and they spread via blood to the lungs and bone. Treatment is by total thyroidectomy (except for tumours <1 cm, which are resectable with a thyroid lobectomy). Prognosis is 70% at 5 years for papillary cancers. Papillary and follicular carcinomas may be TSH-dependent (i.e. the presence of TSH stimulates their growth). For this reason, after thyroid surgery patients take lifelong thyroxine in order to suppress endogenous TSH secretion and reduce the risk of recurrence.

2. I – Riedel thyroiditis

Riedel thyroiditis is characterized by idiopathic fibrosis of the thyroid gland. Patients present with a slow-growing goitre that is firm and irregular, and it is difficult to distinguish this from cancer without a biopsy. Initially, thyroid function tests are normal, but 30% of affected patients will develop hypothyroidism and hypoparathyroidism. Complications of the fibrosis include tracheal/oesophageal compression and recurrent laryngeal nerve palsy. There is no treatment for Riedel thyroiditis, but palliative surgery can be performed if there are compressive symptoms (e.g. dysphagia or stridor).

Bernhard Moritz Riedel, German surgeon (1846–1916).

3. E – Hashimoto thyroiditis

Hashimoto thyroiditis (or chronic thyroiditis) is an autoimmune condition of the thyroid, which most commonly affects women. Patients present with a diffusely enlarged, rubbery goitre. People with Hashimoto thyroiditis typically become hypothyroid, although many are euthyroid in the early stages of the disease. Autoantibodies to thyroid peroxidase (an enzyme required to make thyroxine) may be found. Treatment of Hashimoto thyroiditis is with thyroxine, which improves the goitre as well as the symptoms.

Hakari Hashimoto, Japanese surgeon (1881–1934).

4. K – Toxic multinodular goitre

Multinodular goitres are most common in middle-aged women and often present with an unsightly swelling or dysphagia. In some cases, one nodule in a multinodular goitre will become an autonomous thyroxine-secreting adenoma, resulting in features of hyperthyroidism. This scenario is known as a toxic multinodular goitre, or 'Plummer disease'. Cardiac features, such as atrial fibrillation and palpitations, often predominate in toxic multinodular goitre. Treatment is with radio-iodine or subtotal thyroidectomy. Anti-thyroid medications such as carbimazole have little effect.

Henry Stanley Plummer, American physician (1874–1937).

5. A – Anaplastic carcinoma

This woman has anaplastic carcinoma, as indicated by her advanced age and acute presentation. Anaplastic carcinoma accounts for <5% of thyroid tumours but is the most aggressive. It presents in older patients with a hard, symmetrical, rapidly enlarging goitre. Spread is to lymph nodes and to local structures, for example the trachea (resulting in stridor) and the recurrent laryngeal nerve (leading to hoarseness). There is no effective treatment for anaplastic thyroid tumours, although palliative radiotherapy or debulking surgery can be done if there is tracheal compression. Most patients (>90%) with anaplastic carcinoma are dead within a year.

THEME 9: MANAGEMENT OF SKIN CONDITIONS

1. I – Reassurance

This boy has Peutz–Jeghers syndrome, a condition characterized by multiple bluish-black freckles around the lips, nose, oral mucosa and fingers, as well as multiple gastrointestinal hamartomatous polyps. These polyps are benign and have only a very low malignant potential. The polyps may predispose to gastrointestinal bleeding or intussusception, but, in the asymptomatic patient, reassurance is sufficient.

Johannes Augustinus Peutz, Dutch physician (1886–1957).

Harold Joseph Jeghers, American physician (1904–1990).

2. F – Oral antibiotics

Impetigo is a superficial skin infection caused by staphylococcus or streptococcus. It generally occurs in children and presents with thin-walled blisters that itch and bleed and have a superficial golden-yellow crust. The lesions are caused by a toxic reaction between the microbes and the epidermis. This results in splitting of the superficial epidermis and hence thin-walled blisters. These lesions eventually heal without scarring. Impetigo is contagious and requires treatment. If there are only a few lesions, treatment is with bactericidal ointment, such as fusidic acid. If there are many lesions, topical therapy would be inappropriate, so oral flucloxacillin is given instead.

Impetigo, from Latin *impetere* = to assail; referring to its aggressively contagious nature.

3. G – Surgical debridement and intravenous antibiotics

Necrotizing fasciitis (known as the 'flesh-eating bug') is a deep infection of the skin most often caused by Group A streptococcus (e.g. *Streptococcus pyogenes*). Infection often starts in an area of trauma or surgery. Affected areas become erythematous and swollen and tissue soon becomes necrotic. Patients feel systemically unwell and have high pyrexia. The infection spreads rapidly and the mortality rate is up to 30%. Management is therefore aggressive, with intravenous broad-spectrum antibiotics and extensive surgical debridement of infected tissues to prevent further spread. The surgeon must remove any skin that appears necrotic (necrotic skin will not bleed) back to healthy margin. Without surgery, necrotizing fasciitis is fatal.

4. H – Surgical excision

This man has a sebaceous cyst (also known as an epidermal cyst). Sebaceous cysts arise from hair follicles in any part of the body (especially the scalp, face, ears, back and upper arms) and contain keratin. They are painless and mobile and often have a central punctum. Although they are not attached to the subcutaneous tissues below, sebaceous cysts are fixed to the overlying skin. Sebaceous cysts are benign and can be ignored, but, if the patient is worried about cosmesis, excision is performed.

5. E – Intravenous antibiotics

Erysipelas is a superficial streptococcal infection that is confined to a fascial compartment and is often found in the face or legs. It presents as a painful red swelling (lymphoedema) with a characteristically well-defined edge. An area of broken skin may also be visualized from where the streptococcus has gained entry. Erysipelas is treated initially with 2 days of intravenous antibiotics followed by a 1–2-week oral course. If it is not treated early, then infection can spread deeper and wider to become cellulitis or necrotizing fasciitis. In erysipelas involving the face, spreading infection can result in cavernous sinus thrombosis.

Erysipelas, from Greek *erusi* = red + *pelas* = skin.

THEME 10: NECK LUMPS

1. B – Cervical rib

The lump in the neck along with paraesthesia specifically in the T1 distribution gives a likely diagnosis of a cervical rib. A cervical rib is a congenital overdevelopment of the transverse process of the C7 vertebra. This so-called 'rib' can interfere with the lower roots of the brachial plexus (T1), the sympathetic nerves and the subclavian vessels, causing thoracic outlet syndrome. These structures pass from the thorax to the proximal arm through the inter-scalene triangle. (Inter-scalene triangle is bounded by the anterior scalene muscle anteriorly, the middle scalene muscle posteriorly and the medial surface of the first thoracic rib inferiorly.) If the T1 root of the brachial plexus is affected (as in this scenario), there is pain and paraesthesia in the T1 distribution (medial aspect of the arm) and wasting of the small muscles of the hand (also supplied by T1). Disturbance of the sympathetic nerves results in Horner syndrome (ipsilateral miosis, ptosis, enophthalmos and anhydrosis). If the subclavian artery is pinched by the cervical rib, there will be a stenosis and reduced blood flow to the arm. This becomes apparent on exertion, because, when the arm needs more blood, it will 'steal' it from the vertebral artery (which should supply the brain). Therefore, if the affected arm is exerted, a loss of consciousness may result. This phenomenon is known as the 'subclavian steal syndrome'. Diagnosis of a cervical rib is by X-ray of the cervical spine. Treatment is by excision.

Johann Friedrich Horner, Swedish ophthalmologist (1831–1886).

2. E – Pleomorphic adenoma

A hard, painless mobile lump near the angle of the jaw in a woman of this age, with no evidence of facial nerve involvement, is likely to be a pleomorphic adenoma. The pleomorphic adenoma is the most common benign tumour of the salivary glands. It is most common in the 40s–50s and the only known risk factor is exposure to radiation. The facial nerve is characteristically not involved (if it were, this feature would imply malignancy). Treatment is by excision of the tumour, which has a good prognosis.

3. C – Chemodectoma

A chemodectoma is a tumour of carotid body chemoreceptors arising in the carotid bifurcation. It is usually benign. A chemodectoma presents as a slowly enlarging neck mass that demonstrates a transmitted carotid pulsation. It characteristically mobilizes side to side but not up and down, as the tumour gets caught in the surrounding structures. Pressure on the tumour may cause dizziness and syncope by stimulating vagal tone via the carotid sinus. Diagnosis is by carotid angiogram, which shows a highly vascularized tumour at the carotid bifurcation. Treatment of chemodectomas is by surgical excision.

Syncope, from Greek *syncopa* = to cut short.

4. H – Sternocleidomastoid tumour

Ischaemic contracture of the sternocleidomastoid muscle can occur due to birth trauma and often presents after a few weeks of life with tilting of the head (torticollis) and a painless fibrous mass in the sternocleidomastoid muscle. Treatment is by passive stretching of the muscle, and the condition eventually disappears by the sixth month of life.

Torticollis, from Latin *torti* = twist + *collis* = neck.

5. D – Dermoid cyst

A dermoid cyst is a cyst that is lined by epidermis and lies deep to the skin. Dermoid cysts are usually benign lesions and can occur anywhere in the body. They are caused when skin is forcibly implanted into the subcutaneous tissues by a cut or stab injury. Dermoid cysts can contain other ectodermal tissues such as hair follicles and sebaceous glands. Treatment is by excision.

THEME 11: PAEDIATRIC ORTHOPAEDIC CONDITIONS

1. H – Talipes equinovarus

In talipes equinovarus ('clubfoot'), the foot is inverted and plantarflexed. Talipes is the most common congenital abnormality, occurring in around 1 in 500 births. Half of the cases are bilateral. Clubfoot may be secondary to intrauterine compression (from oligohydramnios) or a neuromuscular disorder (such as spina bifida). This condition must be managed, else the deformity will persist. Options include passive stretching and strapping. If deformity is severe, corrective surgery is required.

Talipes equinovarus, from Latin *talus* = ankle + *pes* = foot + *equinus* = horse-like + *varus* = inward; inward turning of the ankle and foot, like a horse.

2. G – Spontaneous haemarthrosis

Recurrent acute swellings in joints of children may be due to haemophilia. Trivial trauma may result in bleeding into the joint, most commonly the knee, and this is known as haemarthrosis. Haemophilia is an X-linked recessive deficiency of factor VIII or IX. Recurrent haemarthroses result in pain, stiffness and early osteoarthritis.

3. E – Septic arthritis

Septic arthritis should always be considered with the presentation of a hot, swollen, tender joint with a restricted range of movement in the unwell patient. Septic arthritis is an infection within the synovial joint most often caused by *Staphylococcus aureus* infection. It is most common in the hip and knee. Risk factors for developing septic arthritis include being very old or very young, IV drug use, diabetes, and having pre-existing joint complaints. X-ray is normal in the early stages, but ultrasound and joint aspiration should be done to culture organisms. Management of septic arthritis is with surgical washout of the joint and IV antibiotics (e.g. flucloxacillin and benzylpenicillin) until the patient is clinically well, followed by a few weeks of oral antibiotics. Complications of septic arthritis include joint destruction (leading to arthritis), spread of infection to the bone (osteomyelitis) and ankylosis (bony fusion across the joint).

4. B – Genu varus

Genu varus (or bow-legs) is a deformity characterized by medial angulation of the lower leg at the knee (the term 'valgus' describes the opposite deformity). The most common cause of genu varus is rickets, which is a deficiency of vitamin D resulting in a lack of calcium absorption with subsequent skeletal and dental deformities. Another cause of genu varus in children is Blount's disease, where asymmetric growth of the tibial physis results in a progressive varus deformity at the knee (i.e. the lateral part of the tibia grows quicker than the medial side). Blount disease is more common in Scandinavian and Afro-Caribbean children.

The original Latin words *varus* and *valgus* had the opposite meaning to their modern use in medicine. *Varus* meant 'knock-kneed' and *valgus* meant 'bow-legged', because the Latin words actually described the position of the leg at the hip joint rather than at the knee joint. (Latin *genu* = knee.)

Walter Putnam Blount, American orthopaedic surgeon (1900–1992).

5. C – Osgood–Schlatter disease

Osgood–Schlatter disease is a condition characterized by transient inflammation of the growth plate (i.e. osteochondritis of the tibial tuberosity, where the patellar tendon attaches). It is most common in active boys in their early teens. Features include pain and swelling around the tuberosity, which is worse on activity, especially leg extension. Treatment is with rest and analgesia.

Robert Bayley Osgood, American orthopaedic surgeon (1873–1956).
Carl Schlatter, Swiss physician (1864–1934).

THEME 12: GASTROINTESTINAL POLYPS

1. A – Adenomatous polyp

Adenomatous polyps are benign polyps that have the potential to undergo malignant change. Because of this potential, it is important that such polyps be removed. Multiple adenomatous polyps are found in familial adenomatous polyposis (FAP), a condition that predisposes to colorectal cancer. It has an autosomal dominant inheritance pattern. FAP results from a defect in the APC (adenomatous polyposis coli) gene, which is responsible for the apoptosis of cells of the colon. Consequently all patients with FAP will develop colorectal cancer unless treated. Other malignancies associated with FAP include adenocarcinoma of the duodenum and the ampulla of Vater.

Abraham Vater, German anatomist (1684–1751).

2. B – Hamartomatous polyp

The association of circumoral freckling with multiple duodenal polyps is known as Peutz–Jeghers syndrome (PJS), a rare autosomal dominant condition. The polyps are benign hamartomas (a growth that is made up of the same material from which it arises). However, patients with PJS do have an increased (15-fold) risk of developing a gastrointestinal malignancy.

Johannes Laurentius Peutz, Dutch physician (1886–1957).
Harold Joseph Jeghers, American physician (1904–1990).

3. F – Villous adenoma

Villous adenomas are large polyps that look like sea anemones. Villous adenomas secrete mucus and potassium; hence they can present with diarrhoea and features of hypokalaemia (muscle weakness, myalgia and arrhythmias). Of all the rectal polyps, the villous adenoma has the highest potential for malignant change, so it must be removed.

4. E – Pseudopolyp

Pseudopolyps are found with inflammatory bowel disease. When there is an area of oedematous, swollen bowel surrounded by ulcerations, it looks as if the oedema is protruding from the walls of the bowel wall as a polyp. These 'polyps' merely represent swollen bowel mucosa.

5. C – Juvenile polyp

Juvenile polyps affect 1% of children and young adolescents, but can occur at any age. The word juvenile refers to the histological appearance of the polyp and not the patient's age. They look like a cherry on a stalk. Juvenile polyps are always benign. Some may present with fresh, painless bleeding per rectum and others prolapse on defaecation.

Metaplastic polyps usually do not grow to above 5 mm in size and have very little risk of becoming malignant (despite what the name suggests).

THEME 13: FEMORAL NECK FRACTURES

1. B – Cannulated screws

The issue with intracapsularfemoral neck fractures is blood supply. Displacement of the femoral neck will disrupt the blood supply to the femoral head, with resulting avascular necrosis. In a fit and well person under the age of 65 years who presents with a displaced intracapsular fracture, urgent reduction and internal fixation with a cannulated screw is the management of choice. Where possible, the femoral head should be preserved in young individuals.

2. C – Dynamic hip screws

Inter-trochanteric fractures are outside the joint capsule and therefore do not affect the femoral head blood supply. One treatment option for inter-trochanteric fractures is with a dynamic hip screw (DHS). The DHS involves fixing a plate to the lateral aspect of the femoral shaft. A dynamic screw (a type of lag screw) is then sited in the femoral head through a metallic sleeve. Weight bearing causes a dynamic compression of the fracture. The shaft of the lag screw slides down the sleeve maintaining reduction of the fracture as healing occurs. Another treatment option would be fixation with an intra-medullary nail.

3. B – Cannulated screws

The management of undisplaced femoral neck fractures (Garden I and II) requires the insertion of cannulated screws to avoid late displacement and to attempt preservation of the blood supply to the femoral head. There is a risk of avascular necrosis and non-union; if this occurs, a hemiarthroplasty or total hip replacement may be performed at a later date.

4. D – Hemiarthroplasty

This patient presenting with a displaced subcapital (i.e. intracapsular) femoral fracture is not under 65 years and was not previously fit and well. She is at high risk of avascular necrosis and therefore not a candidate for cannulated screws. Displaced femoral neck fractures (Garden III and IV) require a hemiarthroplasty (replacement of the femoral head). The two main types of hemiarthroplasty available are the Thompson's (cemented) and Austin–Moore (non-cemented). There are extremely few occasions whereby patients who have sustained a neck of femur fracture do not undergo surgery. Without surgery, patients have ongoing pain and are immobile. For the very old and frail, an uncemented hemiarthroplasty represents a favourable surgical option as the operative risk is reduced (no cement and shorter anaesthetic time).

5. F – Total hip replacement

This man over 65 years has a displaced femoral neck fracture affecting the blood supply to the femoral head. Normally this would be managed with a hemiarthroplasty, but, because this patient has preceding osteoarthritis, a total hip replacement would be more appropriate, as this would also alleviate arthritic symptoms.

THEME 14: DIAGNOSIS OF GROIN LUMPS

1. L – Varicocele

This man has a swelling that does not transilluminate, disappears on lying down but does not have a cough impulse. This is characteristic of a varicocele. (An indirect inguinal hernia would exhibit a cough impulse.) The term 'varicocele' describes varicosities in the pampiniform venous plexus, the network of veins that drains the testicle. It usually occurs on the left side and is present in 10% of males. Patients present with a scrotal swelling on standing that feels like a 'bag of worms', and may experience a heavy, dragging sensation. Varicoceles are usually harmless, but have been associated with defective spermatogenesis rendering some patients subfertile (although this is a contentious issue). Varicoceles can be diagnosed by ultrasound, which shows venous dilatation greater than 2 mm. Good practice would be to include an ultrasound of the left kidney as well. Unlike the right testicle that drains directly into the inferior vena cava, the left testicle drains via the left renal vein. Cancers of the left kidney can present with a left-sided varicocele, as the presence of the tumour can impair venous return from the testicle. Management is by reassurance and wearing supportive underwear. If a patient desires treatment then radiological embolization of the left testicular vein, or ligation and division of the testicular veins, can be performed.

2. C – Hydrocele

A hydrocele is a collection of serous fluid in the tunica vaginalis, a membrane that covers the testis. Hydroceles can be primary or secondary to an underlying cause. Primary hydroceles (as in this case) are tense, painless, fluctuant swellings that transilluminate. Because the fluid surrounds the testicle, the underlying testis is not palpable. The epididymis above can be felt as a separate structure. Primary hydroceles are benign, but can be surgically excised if desired. (Simple aspiration of the cyst will result in reaccumulation of fluid.) A secondary hydrocele can occur when the membranous sac around the testis becomes filled with exudates secondary to tumours or inflammation of the underlying testis or epididymis. Secondary hydroceles are usually small and lax. An ultrasound scan should be performed in all adults presenting with a hydrocele to exclude an underlying tumour. Secondary hydroceles require treatment of the underlying condition.

3. G – Sebaceous cyst

Sebaceous cysts (or epidermal cysts) are the most common cystic skin lesion. They can occur on the scrotum (as well as the scalp, ears, back, face and chest) and may only be noticed if they become infected. Sebaceous cysts are soft swellings that are fixed to the overlying skin but not to the tissues underneath. A central punctum may be visible through which a cheesy foul-smelling fluid may discharge if the cyst becomes infected. They are the result of proliferation of epidermoid cells within the dermis. Treatment is by reassurance or excision.

4. D – Mumps orchitis

The association of a swollen, painful testicle with viral meningitis points to mumps orchitis as the best answer. Mumps is caused by a paramyxovirus infection that is spread by saliva droplets and can involve multiple organs through haematogenous spread. It most commonly occurs in children. As well as constitutional symptoms, patients develop inflammation of the parotid glands (parotitis). Recognized complications of mumps include meningitis, encephalitis, pancreatitis and orchitis, from which there is a small risk of sterility. The incidence of mumps has been drastically reduced by routine administration of the MMR (measles, mumps, rubella) vaccine.

5. F – Saphena varix

A saphena varix is a dilatation of the long saphenous vein that occurs due to valvular incompetence at the saphenofemoral junction (the confluence of the great saphenous vein and the femoral vein) which is located an inch below and lateral to the pubic tubercle, just medial to the femoral pulse. A saphena varix often has a bluish tinge, is soft and compressible, disappears on lying down, has a cough impulse and exhibits a fluid thrill when the long saphenous vein is tapped distally (Schwart test). It is often associated with varicosities elsewhere in the saphenous system.

THEME 15: CLASSIFICATION OF HERNIAS

A hernia is defined as the protrusion of a viscus or part of a viscus through an abnormal opening in the walls of its containing cavity.

Hernia, from Greek *hernios* = to sprout forth.

1. D – Reducible

This man has an indirect inguinal hernia that is reducible. That means that the contents of the hernia can be returned to the abdomen either by lying down or by manual pressure. Reducible hernias also exhibit an expansile cough impulse.

2. A – Incarcerated

This patient has an incarcerated incisional hernia. In the context of hernias, it describes the inability of the hernia to be reduced back to its normal position (i.e. the hernia is locked in its abnormal position). A hernia becomes incarcerated if adhesions develop between the hernial sac and its contents. The contents of an irreducible hernia cannot be returned to the abdomen and there is no cough impulse, but the patient is asymptomatic. Incarcerated hernias predispose to strangulation.

Incarcerate, from the Latin *in* = in + *carcer* = prison.

3. G – Strangulated

This woman has features of an obstruction (vomiting and colicky abdominal pain) along with a painful, erythematous hernia. This suggests a diagnosis of strangulation. A hernia strangulates when it twists upon itself and interferes with its blood supply. Initially, venous return is obstructed, and the oedema that results eventually cuts off the arterial supply. Ischaemia and necrosis follow, with gangrene developing within 6 hours. On examination, a strangulated hernia will be irreducible, tender, erythematous and warm. Femoral hernias (as in this scenario) are very likely to strangulate due to their narrow neck. Treatment involves fluid resuscitation and urgent surgery.

An obstructed hernia is an irreducible hernia that contains obstructed bowel without interference to the blood supply. The symptoms (i.e. colicky abdominal pain, vomiting, distension and constipation) are less severe and of more gradual onset compared with strangulation. Obstruction usually progresses to strangulation.

4. E – Richter

A Richter hernia describes strangulation of one sidewall of the bowel within a hernial sac (unlike a strangulated hernia, where there is strangulation of the entire lumen of the bowel). This results in the features of strangulation (pain and erythema with a risk of gangrene and perforation) without characteristics of obstruction.

August Richter, German surgeon (1742–1812).

5. C – Perforated

This woman presents with features of peritonitis, namely a painful, rigid, 'board-like' abdomen with pyrexia, tachycardia and vomiting. This, along with an erythematous hernia, points to a diagnosis of hernial perforation following strangulation. An urgent laparotomy is required along with antibiotics.

THEME 16: INVESTIGATION OF VASCULAR DISEASE

1. D – Duplex Doppler ultrasound

This woman presents with sudden-onset weakness that resolves within 24 hours, characteristic of a transient ischaemic attack (TIA). TIAs are often caused by atheromatous emboli from the carotid arteries and can present with transient weakness, dizziness or visual disturbance (amaurosis fugax). Risk factors include smoking, hypertension, diabetes and hypercholesterolaemia. TIAs are themselves an important risk factor for subsequent disabling stroke (there is a 13-fold increased risk in the next year). People presenting with a TIA should be investigated for underlying carotid stenosis, as patients with a stenosis greater than 60% may benefit from a carotid endarterectomy. Other indications for carotid endarterectomy include 70% stenosis if the patient is asymptomatic. The best screening investigation for assessing the degree of carotid stenosis is Doppler ultrasound.

The Duplex Doppler ultrasound has two aspects (hence 'duplex'). First, a grey-scale ultrasound is used to visualize the vessels and the degree of stenosis in millimetres. Then the Doppler feature is used to measure the blood velocity through the vessel, which is proportional to the degree of stenosis of the vessel (i.e. the greater the velocity, the greater the stenosis). Ultrasound has the advantage over angiography as it is non-invasive and safe as a screening tool. For patients who are suitable for surgery, preoperative angiography can be performed to more accurately determine the position of the stenosis. Angiography does carry a risk of TIA (3%) and stroke (0.1%) during the procedure. Note that the presence of a carotid bruit on examination bears no relationship to the severity of stenosis, as very tight stenoses may be silent.

Christian Doppler, Austrian physicist (1803–1853). Described the Doppler effect – the apparent change in the frequency and wavelength of a wave that is perceived by an observer moving relative to the source of the wave.

2. A – Ankle–brachial pressure index

This man presents with features of peripheral vascular disease (PVD). The best way to confirm the presence of PVD is by using the ankle–brachial pressure index (ABPI). The blood pressure in the foot should be similar to that in the arm. In peripheral vascular disease, the pressure in the foot is reduced due to atherosclerotic disease. The foot artery pressure is measured by placing a blood pressure cuff around the calf. A hand-held Doppler is used to find the dorsalis pedis or posterior tibial pulse and the cuff is inflated until the Doppler signal disappears (this point is the foot artery occlusion pressure). The ABPI is then calculated by dividing the foot artery occlusion pressure by the brachial systolic pressure. The dorsalis pedis pulse should be found just lateral to extensor hallucis longus and dosalis pedis can be found in the groove between the medial malleolus and the Achilles tendon.

An ABPI of 0.9–1.1 is considered the normal range. Mild ischaemia is denoted by an ABPI of 0.7–0.9 and moderate ischaemia by an ABPI of 0.4–0.7. Severe (critical) limb ischaemia is accompanied by an ABPI < 0.4. Critical limb ischaemia is defined as rest pain lasting over 2 weeks, with or without ulceration or gangrene. An ABPI > 1.1 (i.e. the foot artery occlusion pressure is significantly larger than the brachial systolic pressure) implies the presence of calcified or incompressible vessels, which occur with diabetes or renal failure.

The ABPI, along with the clinical symptoms, can be used as a guide to further investigation and management. Mild ischaemia is managed with conservative measures and best medical therapy (statin, aspirin, etc.). Moderate ischaemia will need vascular outpatient referral with further imaging (duplex scan and/or angiogram). Severe symptoms and critical limb ischaemia require urgent vascular surgical or radiological intervention.

3. E – Hand-held Doppler

There are many clinical examination techniques used to help determine the sites of venous incompetence in varicose veins, but the best of these is use of a hand-held Doppler. The probe is placed over the site of potential incompetence and the leg distal to the probe is squeezed. A 'whoosh' sound is heard as blood is squeezed through the vein and, on letting go of the leg, another 'whoosh' is heard as blood rushes back through the incompetent section of vein. More formal investigation of varicose veins can be done by duplex scanning or venography. Venography is an invasive investigation where radio-opaque dye is infused into the veins whilst X-rays are taken.

4. D – Duplex Doppler ultrasound

This patient has moderate peripheral vascular disease. The subsequent operative management of his leg depends on the underlying arterial lesions, and the first investigation that should be performed to determine these is duplex ultrasonography. The use of contrast arteriography should only be requested if the duplex scanning yields equivocal results or if there is a plan to proceed to revascularization. In contrast angiography, a radio-opaque dye is injected into a vessel and X-rays are taken of the limb. Surgical management options for peripheral vascular disease include angioplasty, arterial reconstruction and amputation.

5. G – No investigation required

This man presents with features strongly suggesting a ruptured abdominal aortic aneurysm (AAA). Ruptured AAAs have a high morbidity and mortality and, unless the diagnosis is in doubt, urgent surgery is required. Had the patient been more haemodynamically stable (suggesting a leaking aneurysm, rather than rupture), an abdominal ultrasound would quickly aid diagnosis.

Practice Paper 3: Questions

THEME 1: UPPER GASTROINTESTINAL HAEMORRHAGE

Options

A. Aorto-enteric fistula
B. Carcinoma of the stomach
C. Carcinoma of the oesophagus
D. Epistaxis
E. Haemoptysis
F. Mallory–Weiss tear
G. Oesophageal varices
H. Peptic ulceration
I. Boerhaave syndrome

For each of the following people presenting with bleeding, select the most appropriate diagnosis. Each option may be used once, more than once or not at all.

1. A 62-year-old man is brought to the emergency department after vomiting large amounts of fresh blood. On examination, he is drowsy with a heart rate of 120/min and blood pressure of 92/50 mmHg. An urgent full blood count shows haemoglobin 6.9 g/dL, platelets 160 × 10^9/L, mean cell volume 106 and INR 2.3.
2. A 25-year-old man presents with three episodes of vomiting that contained altered blood. He has recently started a busy job that he finds stressful and he has not had time to eat well. In addition, he complains of a 6-month history of upper abdominal pain that is relieved by eating and for which he takes ibuprofen.
3. A 19-year-old student presents with blood-stained vomiting. He was on a pub crawl last night and spent the latter hours of the night vomiting and retching over a bucket.
4. A 59-year-old man presents vomiting copious amounts of fresh blood. On examination, his pulse is 138/min and blood pressure 68/42 mmHg. A per rectum exam demonstrates melaena and fresh blood. Apart from an abdominal aortic aneurysm repair last year, he denies any medical history.
5. An 83-year-old man attends the emergency department after vomiting small amounts of fresh blood. He complains of a 3-month history

of aching pain in his epigastrium and a poor appetite, saying he lost over 2 stone in this period. The patient denies difficulty swallowing. On examination, you find enlarged supraclavicular lymph nodes.

THEME 2: AIRWAY MANAGEMENT

Options

A. Bag and mask
B. Double-lumen cuffed endotracheal tube
C. Head tilt chin lift
D. Nasopharyngeal airway
E. Needle cricothyroidotomy
F. Oropharyngeal airway
G. Single-lumen cuffed endotracheal tube
H. Single-lumen uncuffed endotracheal tube
I. Surgical tracheostomy

For each of the following presentations, select the next most appropriate step in management of the airway. Each option may be used once, more than once or not at all.

1. You are called to see a 67-year-old woman who has oxygen saturations of 70%. She has just returned from theatre following an elective cholecystectomy. The patient is drowsy and, as you approach, you hear inspiratory grunting.
2. A 56-year-old man is being prepared to undergo an elective liver resection for a primary hepatocellular carcinoma.
3. A 62-year-old man is being prepared to undergo an elective thoracic aortic aneurysm repair.
4. A 6-year-old child was brought to the emergency department after being involved in a fire at home. There is soot around his nose and there is a marked respiratory effort. His respiratory rate is 36/min and his oxygen saturations read 88% on 35% oxygen.
5. A 28-year-old man is rushed to hospital following a road traffic accident. He has severe injuries to his head and neck. The patient goes into respiratory arrest and two attempts at endotracheal intubation fail.

THEME 3: PANCREATIC TUMOURS

Options

A. Gastrinoma
B. Glucagonoma
C. Insulinoma
D. Non-secreting islet cell tumour
E. Somatostatinoma
F. VIPoma

For each of the following presentations, select the most appropriate diagnosis. Each option may be used once, more than once or not at all.

1. A 42-year-old man presents with episodes of faintness and tiredness. The symptoms are worse after exercise and are relieved by eating. On examination, he is pale and sweaty.
2. A 48-year-old woman presents with a 4-week history of watery diarrhoea, having up to 15 episodes a day. On examination, she is severely dehydrated and her blood results show Na 134 mmol/L, K 2.9 mmol/L, urea 13 mmol/L and creatinine 132 μmol/L. A stool culture is negative.
3. A 38-year-old woman presents with a 2-week history of thirst and urinary frequency. She admits to losing 3 kg in weight over this period. On examination, she has an erythematous, blistering rash over her buttocks.
4. A 54-year-old man presents with coffee-ground vomiting. He describes suffering with intermittent epigastric pain and diarrhoea over the last month. An endoscopy is ordered and determines the presence of multiple, large ulcers and erosions over the stomach, duodenum and proximal jejunum.
5. A 48-year-old woman presents with a long history of foul-smelling, bulky stools. These episodes are getting more frequent and more severe. She also admits to drinking lots and passing large amounts of dilute urine. On examination, the patient appears thin and wasted, but there is no other abnormality.

THEME 4: ENDOCRINE DISORDERS

Options

A. Acromegaly
B. Addison disease
C. Carcinoid tumour
D. Congenital adrenal hyperplasia
E. Conn syndrome
F. Cushing syndrome
G. Hyperparathyroidism
H. Hypoparathyroidism
I. Multiple endocrine neoplasia type 1
J. Multiple endocrine neoplasia type 2
K. Multiple endocrine neoplasia type 3
L. Nelson syndrome
M. Phaeochromocytoma

For each of the following people with endocrine disorders, select the most likely diagnosis. Each option may be used once, more than once or not at all.

1. A 54-year-old man presents to the clinic complaining of paraesthesia in both of his hands. He has also noticed a slight change in his appearance, mentioning that his nose looks bigger. He has a past medical history of hypertension and diabetes. On examination, you find abnormal sensation in the lateral three and a half digits of the hands.
2. A 52-year-old woman presents with increased skin pigmentation. She denies using sunbeds or sunbathing. You note that she has been treated for Cushing disease in the past.
3. A 34-year-old man presents to the emergency department with epigastric pain. He admits having brain surgery in the past for a tumour that caused him to produce milk. While you are taking a history, the patient suffers a large haematemesis, and an urgent endoscopy is arranged. The endoscopist notes multiple large ulcers throughout the stomach, duodenum and jejunum.
4. A 48-year-old woman presents with frequency of urine and excessive thirst. She also complains of occasional muscle cramps. She has history of hypertension but is not on any regular medication. Capillary glucose is 4.2 mmol/L, and routine blood tests show sodium 148 mmol/L and potassium 3.2 mmol/L.
5. A 24-year-old man presents to his general practitioner with a lump in his neck that has been growing slowly over a few weeks. On examination, you note that he is tall and has long digits. He tells you that his father died of adrenal cancer.

THEME 5: MANAGEMENT OF ABDOMINAL PAIN

Options

A. Azathioprine
B. Augmentin
C. Cefuroxime and metronidazole
D. Lansoprazole alone
E. Metoclopramide
F. Ofloxacin and metronidazole
G. Omeprazole, clarithromycin and metronidazole
H. Opioid analgesia alone
I. Steroids

For each of the following people presenting with abdominal pain, select the most appropriate management. Each option may be used once, more than once or not at all.

1. A 72-year-old woman presents with a 2-day history of lower abdominal pain, vomiting and diarrhoea. Her abdomen is tender with guarding in the left iliac fossa and her temperature is 38.2°C.
2. A 42-year-old woman complains of a long history of abdominal bloating. She feels full after eating small amounts and tends to vomit soon after eating. She has a medical history of diabetes and rheumatoid arthritis.

An endoscopy shows a dilated stomach with some stale food in it. There is no evidence of ulceration or obstruction.

3. A 32-year-old man attends the emergency department with a short history of epigastric pain and vomiting. On examination, there is some epigastric tenderness but no guarding. An upper endoscopy is performed and shows evidence of inflammation and ulceration in the stomach. A CLO test comes back positive.
4. A 21-year-old woman presents with a 2-day history of lower abdominal pain, dysuria and vomiting. On examination, there is guarding in the left iliac fossa. A per rectum exam is normal but there is evidence of a yellow vaginal discharge.
5. A 25-year-old woman with previously well-controlled ulcerative colitis presents with a 2-day history of severe lower abdominal pain and bloody diarrhoea. She is pyrexial on examination.

THEME 6: SKIN LESIONS

Options

A. Cellulitis
B. Erysipelas
C. Ganglion
D. Granuloma annulare
E. Impetigo
F. Kaposi's sarcoma
G. Necrotizing fasciitis
H. Neurofibroma
I. Pyogenic granuloma
J. Sebaceous cyst
K. Seborrhoeic keratosis
L. Thrombophlebitis

For each of the following people presenting with skin lesions, select the most likely diagnosis. Each option may be used once, more than once or not at all.

1. A 35-year-old man who has a history of end-stage renal failure managed by transplant presents with multiple painless purple palpable lesions that have gradually appeared over the last few weeks. These lesions are found all over his body.
2. A 34-year-old woman attends the diabetes clinic for a check-up. She shows the doctor a lesion on the back of her hand that has appeared recently. They do not cause any problems, but she was just curious. On examination, the lesion is made up of reddish bumps that are arranged in a ring.
3. A 28-year-old man presents with a bright-red nodule on the end of his index finger that bleeds easily. This lesion has grown rapidly in the last week and is now 1 cm in diameter.

4. A 15-year-old girl presents with multiple lumps on her arms and trunk. On examination, the lesions feel firm and rubbery and the patient reports some tingling on palpation.
5. A 45-year-old man who is in hospital following an elective cholecystectomy shows the house officer an area of erythema around his intravenous cannula site. On examination, the area is also swollen and warm, with some superficial blistering. The patient has a temperature of 38.5°C and feels unwell.

THEME 7: CONDITIONS OF THE NOSE

Options

A. Acute ethmoid sinusitis
B. Acute frontal sinusitis
C. Acute maxillary sinusitis
D. Allergic rhinitis
E. Chemical irritation
F. Chronic sinusitis
G. Foreign body
H. Hypertensive epistaxis
I. Non-accidental injury
J. Non-allergic rhinitis
K. Spontaneous epistaxis
L. Wegener's granulomatosis

For each of the following presentations, select the most likely diagnosis. Each option may be used once, more than once or not at all.

1. An 18-month-old boy presents to the general practitioner with a 3-week history of a blood-stained, foul-smelling discharge from the left nostril. His mother denies any history of trauma to the area. On examination, the membrane of the left nasal canal is inflamed. Examination of the opposite side shows no abnormality.
2. A 7-year-old boy is brought to the doctor by his mother with a long history of intermittent nose bleeds. The bleeding occurs spontaneously and lasts around 10 minutes each time. He is well in between episodes. Examination is unremarkable.
3. A 17-year-old girl presents with a 1-week history of headache and facial pain that is worse on coughing. She is worried about failing her advanced level modules as she has already had 2 weeks off school with a cold. On examination, she is tender over the left cheek, but there is no obvious swelling.
4. A 32-year-old man of no fixed abode is referred to the ENT specialist with a 12-month history of intermittent epistaxis. He denies any other symptoms. On examination, there is a small defect in the nasal septum and some evidence of recent bleeding.

5. A 23-year-old man presents with a 2-month history of a watery nasal discharge associated with sneezing attacks and eye irritation. This is worse when he is outdoors. He has never suffered these symptoms in the past. On examination, there is no evidence of nasal polyps.

THEME 8: PAEDIATRIC ORTHOPAEDIC CONDITIONS

Options

A. Developmental dysplasia of the hip
B. Genu varus
C. Osgood–Schlatter disease
D. Perthes disease
E. Septic arthritis
F. Slipped upper femoral epiphysis
G. Spontaneous haemarthrosis
H. Still disease
I. Talipes equinovarus
J. Transient synovitis

For each of the following presentations, select the most likely diagnosis. Each option may be used once, more than once or not at all.

1. A 13-year-old boy is brought to the emergency department with a limp. This developed after he was tackled playing football last week, and he is now complaining of pain in his left hip and knee. On examination, he is apyrexial and appears overweight. His left leg is externally rotated and shorter than the right.
2. A 9-year-old boy is taken to his general practitioner by his mother with increasing pain on walking. On examination, he is apyrexial and movement in his left hip is restricted because of pain. An X-ray of the left femoral head shows it to be dense and irregular.
3. A 10-year-old girl is brought to the emergency department with sudden-onset right hip pain that started 2 days ago and occurred at rest. The pain caused some difficulty walking, although there is no pain at rest. Her mother is worried, as the girl has already missed a week of school for a cold. On examination, she is apyrexial, but examination of the hip is difficult due to pain. An X-ray of the right femoral head shows no obvious abnormality.
4. A 6-week-old baby girl is visited by the community midwife for her neonatal check. The midwife notices that there is limited abduction in her right leg. As the midwife abducts the girl's right leg while placing anterior pressure on it, she feels a 'clunk'.
5. A 4-year-old girl presents with a long-standing history of a limp. She has also been feeling unwell and has an intermittent fever. On examination, the girl is pyrexial and you notice a pink rash on her legs. There is tenderness in both hips and knees.

THEME 9: MANAGEMENT OF PROSTATE DISEASE

Options

A. Active surveillance
B. Brachytherapy
C. Doxazosin
D. External-beam radiotherapy
E. Finasteride
F. Radical prostatectomy
G. Transurethral resection of prostate

For each of the following scenarios, select the most appropriate management. Each option may be used once, more than once or not at all.

1. An 87-year-old man has a transrectal ultrasound-guided biopsy following admission for acute urinary retention. Histology shows a T1 prostate cancer.
2. A 68-year-old man with known metastatic prostate cancer presents with worsening bony pain in his left hip. He is currently on a course of hormonal treatment.
3. A 57-year-old man is diagnosed with a T2 prostate cancer. He expresses a wish to have curative therapy but mentions that he would like to reduce the risk of developing impotence as a result of therapy.
4. A 63-year-old man presents with a 6-month history of poor stream and dribbling at the end of micturation, which is bothering him. He is found to have smooth prostatic enlargement on digital rectal examination. His PSA is 7.5 ng/mL.
5. A 58-year-old man who has benign prostatic hyperplasia has been treated with finasteride for over a year. He presents to the clinic because he has found no benefit in his symptoms since being started on medical management.

THEME 10: STATISTICS

Options

A. 17%
B. 25%
C. 50%
D. 67%
E. 75%
F. 83%
G. 1.5
H. 2.5
I. 3.0
J. 4.5
K. 6.0

A new blood test is being developed to help detect the presence of colorectal liver metastases. In a trial, 500 patients have been tested. The trial produces 200 positive results and 300 negative results. Of the 200 positive results, 50 are false positives. Of the 300 negative results, 50 are false negatives.
What is the:

1. Sensitivity
2. Specificity
3. Positive predictive value
4. Negative predictive value
5. Likelihood ratio

THEME 11: KNEE INJURIES

Options

A. Anterior cruciate injury
B. Lateral collateral injury
C. Lateral meniscus tear
D. Medial collateral injury
E. Medial meniscus tear
F. Osteoarthritis
G. Osteochondritis dessicans
H. Patellar fracture
I. Posterior cruciate injury
J. Rheumatoid arthritis
K. Tibial plateau fracture

For each of the following people presenting with knee problems, select the most likely diagnosis. Each option may be used once, more than once or not at all.

1. A 65-year-old man tripped over while walking on a cobbled street and landed on his left knee. On examination, his left knee is swollen and painful. Although the patient is able to walk with help, he cannot straight leg raise.
2. A 22-year-old man was tackled awkwardly during a football match. He says he felt his right knee pop, after which it swelled immediately. He was unable to complete the game. On examination, Lachman test is positive.
3. A 36-year-old woman was hit by a car as she was walking across a zebra crossing. She is now unable to weight-bear on the affected knee. On examination, her knee is painful, bruised and swollen.
4. A 32-year-old man twisted his knee while skiing. Although his knee was painful, he managed to complete the run. By the next morning, his knee was visibly swollen. On examination, you find that he cannot flex or extend his knee fully. He is also tender over the medial joint line.

5. A 34-year-old man was kicked in the knee while playing football. He describes his right knee being hit from the right-hand side. Since the tackle, he has been unable to weight-bear and feels as if his knee is very unsteady. On examination, his knee is tender but not swollen. There is considerable laxity on valgus stress.

THEME 12: MANAGEMENT OF ANORECTAL CONDITIONS

Options

A. DeLorme procedure
B. Diltiazem cream
C. Excision of fistula
D. Incision and drainage
E. Injection sclerotherapy
F. Laying open of the fistula tract
G. Lord's procedure
H. Seton insertion
I. Surgical haemorrhoidectomy

For each of the following presentations, select the most appropriate management. Each option may be used once, more than once or not at all.

1. A 56-year-old woman presents with a history of fresh rectal bleeding after defaecation. On examination, with a proctoscope, haemorrhoids are seen within the anal canal. The patient denies any prolapse of these haemorrhoids.
2. A 71-year-old woman presents with pruritus ani. On examination, she has an obvious prolapsed rectum.
3. A 22-year-old female with known inflammatory bowel disease presents with a constant discharge from the anus. On examination, two external openings are seen at the posterior margin of the anus, both of which are discharging faeculent material. An MRI scan shows a high-lying anal fistula that passes through the puborectalis muscle.
4. A 42-year-old man presents with a 2-day history of pain around his anus, difficulty sitting down and fever. On examination, there is a 1 cm tender, erythematous lump adjacent to the anal margin. No other abnormality is evident.
5. A 34-year-old woman presents with a 7-day history of severe stinging pain in the anus on defaecation, associated with fresh blood on the toilet paper. Examination reveals a tight anal tone and a lone skin tag on the posterior margin of the anus.

THEME 13: UPPER LIMB NERVE LESIONS

Options

A. Accessory nerve
B. Axillary nerve

C. Distal median nerve
D. Distal ulnar nerve
E. Long thoracic nerve
F. Lower brachial plexus
G. Proximal median nerve
H. Proximal ulnar nerve
I. Radial nerve
J. Upper brachial plexus

For each of the following people presenting with neurological problems, select the most likely nerve involved. Each option may be used once, more than once or not at all.

1. A 34-year-old man presents with severe shoulder pain following a tackle during a rugby match. On examination, the contour of the affected shoulder is flattened and the humeral head is palpable in the infraclavicular fossa. There is also sensory loss at the upper lateral aspect of the arm.
2. A 12-year-old boy attends an orthopaedics follow-up clinic after a supracondylar fracture of the left elbow. The surgeon notes that there is hyperextension of the metacarpophalangeal joints of the fourth and fifth digits, with flexion of the interphalangeal joints.
3. A 57-year-old woman attends a follow-up clinic after a right mastectomy for invasive breast cancer. Her husband has pointed out that her right shoulder blade occasionally sticks out more than the left. On examination, there is no evidence of sensory loss.
4. A 37-year-old man was involved in a motorcycle accident 3 months ago and has since been undergoing rehabilitation for extensive injuries. He turns up to a rehabilitation clinic, where you notice that he has hyperextension of all his metacarpophalangeal joints with interphalangeal flexion. On examination, you note a lack of sensation along the ulnar border of the forearm.
5. A 23-year-old man who recently had a cystic hygroma removed attends for follow-up. He complains of pain in the left side of his neck. On examination, he is unable to shrug his left shoulder.

THEME 14: ANATOMY OF HERNIAS

Options

A. Amyand
B. Gluteal
C. Littre
D. Lumbar
E. Maydl
F. Obturator
G. Pantaloon
H. Sciatic

For each of the following descriptions of hernia, choose the correct name. Each option may be used once, more than once or not at all.

1. A hernia that has two parts, each either side of the inferior epigastric artery.
2. A hernia that passes through the greater sciatic foramen.
3. A hernia that contains a 'W' loop of intestine within its sac.
4. A hernia that arises from the triangle of Petit.
5. A hernia that contains the appendix within its sac.

THEME 15: MANAGEMENT OF COMMON FRACTURES

Options

A. Analgesia alone
B. Broad arm sling
C. Dynamic hip screw
D. Hemiarthroplasty
E. Intramedullary nail
F. Manipulation under anaesthesia
G. Open reduction and internal fixation
H. Plaster cast
I. Traction

For each of the following common fractures, select the most appropriate management. Each option may be used once, more than once or not at all.

1. A 65-year-old woman presents following a fall on an outstretched hand. She is found to have a fracture of the distal radius with dorsal displacement of the distal fragment.
2. A 26-year-old man presents to the emergency department after falling off his bike onto his shoulder. He is holding his right arm. An X-ray confirms an undisplaced fracture of the clavicle.
3. A 75-year-old woman presents with an intertrochanteric fracture of the left femur after a fall.
4. A 21-year-old woman sustains a fracture of the shaft of the humerus during a road traffic accident. There is only mild displacement of the fragments.
5. An 18-year-old female student nurse presents with pain in the second toe that has been present for 4 days. She has recently started her clinical placements. An X-ray of the foot shows a hairline fracture of the second metatarsal.

THEME 16: DIAGNOSIS OF VASCULAR DISEASE

Options

A. Buerger disease
B. Deep vein thrombosis (DVT)

C. Embolus
D. Intermittent claudication
E. Klippel–Trénaunay syndrome
F. Raynaud disease
G. Ruptured Baker cyst
H. Spinal stenosis
I. Sturge–Weber syndrome
J. Superficial thrombophlebitis
K. Takayasu arteritis

For each of the following people presenting with vascular disease, select the most appropriate diagnosis. Each option may be used once, more than once or not at all.

1. A 30-year-old woman presents with bilateral arm pain on exertion, which is gradually worsening in severity, and transient visual disturbance. She also complains of feeling unwell and having fever and night sweats. Peripheral and central neurological examinations were normal, but no upper or lower limb pulses are palpable.
2. A 60-year-old man is in hospital following a liver resection 3 days previously. You are called to see him as he is complaining of pain in his right calf. On examination, the calf is swollen, tender and erythematous. Distal pulses are palpable and there is no loss in sensation.
3. A 5-year-old child is brought to the general practitioner by his mother as he is having difficulty walking. On examination, his right leg appears deformed. It is longer and wider than the left, with varicose veins and two purple macules on the thigh.
4. A 46-year-old woman presents to the emergency department with painful, white fingers. The ring and little fingers of her right hand look pale and feel cold, although the other digits are unaffected and distal pulses are present.
5. A 57-year-old man presents with leg cramps on the right side when he walks. The pain is relieved by rest. On examination, there is no evidence of ulceration, but the pedal pulses on the right side are not as strong as those on the left.

Practice Paper 3: Answers

THEME 1: UPPER GASTROINTESTINAL HAEMORRHAGE

1. G – Oesophageal varices

This man is vomiting massive amounts of fresh blood. A raised mean cell volume and deranged clotting with the clinical presentation suggest liver disease secondary to excess alcohol consumption. Oesophageal varices occur as a result of portal hypertension, which in this case is likely to be due to a cirrhotic liver (the most common cause). Portal hypertension results in the formation of collateral vessels between the portal and systemic circulations as follows: between the left gastric and oesophageal veins (→ oesophageal varices), from the obliterated umbilical vein (this forms the superior margin of the falciform ligament) to the superior and inferior epigastric veins (→ caput medusae), between the superior and inferior rectal veins (→ anal canal varices), and finally in the retroperitoneum. Other features of portal hypertension are splenomegaly and ascites. The management of variceal bleeding is by immediate fluid and blood resuscitation, with correction of any clotting abnormalities, followed by an urgent endoscopy to control the bleeding. This can be achieved with clipping, banding, or injection of sclerosants or adrenaline.

2. H – Peptic ulceration

The history of epigastric pain that is relieved by eating is a classic presentation of a duodenal ulcer. A peptic ulcer is defined as an ulcer that occurs in the lower oesophagus, stomach or small intestine. Erosions are more superficial than ulcers in that erosions do not penetrate the muscle layer. Ulcers *do* penetrate the muscle layer. Peptic ulcers can be divided into acute and chronic. The most common causes of acute peptic ulcers are *Helicobacter pylori* infection, which accounts for 80% of cases, and NSAID use. NSAIDs cause peptic ulceration by inhibiting the synthesis of prostaglandins that usually protect the gastric mucosa from acid attack. Other causes of acute peptic ulceration include operations, steroid use and stress. Cushing ulcers arise following head injury. Curling ulcers arise secondary to severe burns. Eighty percent of chronic peptic ulcers occur in the duodenum, mostly on the anterior wall of the first part of the duodenum. They are more common in males in their 30s. Chronic gastric ulcers are usually situated on the lesser curvature. Again they are more common in males, but in a slightly older age group.

The features of peptic ulcer disease include intermittent epigastric pain that can radiate to the back. The pain may start *immediately* after eating, but it usually starts *2 hours* after eating. Because the pain often starts so long after eating, patients commonly think that the pain is brought about by *not* eating. This is why people complain of 'hunger pain'. In reality, you cannot tell if an ulcer is gastric or duodenal based on the time relationship between eating and the onset of pain. The pain of peptic ulcers tends to be worse with spicy foods but is relieved by milk and alkalis. The best investigation for peptic ulcers is an upper GI endoscopy with multiple biopsies of the ulcer to exclude malignant transformation within these lesions. Management of peptic ulcers is conservative (avoid smoking, stress, NSAIDs and aspirin) and medical. The best medical management for increased acid secretion is by the use of proton pump inhibitors (PPIs). PPIs irreversibly inhibit the action of the hydrogen/potassium ion ATPase pump of the parietal cells of the stomach. These drugs achieve achlorhydria (low levels of acid production) within a few days, and ulcers heal within 2 months. However, if PPI use is withdrawn then ulcers can re-develop. The reason why PPIs are so effective is due to the fact that they act at the terminal step of gastric acid secretion. Consequently, surgical intervention is rarely required for peptic ulcer disease.

3. F – Mallory-Weiss tear

A Mallory-Weiss tear is a superficial tear in the mucosa of the lower oesophagus resulting in a bleed. The tear can be caused by severe coughing, retching or vomiting. Definitive diagnosis is by endoscopy. In most cases, bleeding settles spontaneously after 48 hours.

George Kenneth Mallory, American pathologist (1900–1986).
Soma Weiss, Hungarian physician (1898–1942).

4. A – Aorto-enteric fistula

An aorto-enteric fistula is a rare but recognized complication of abdominal aortic aneurysm repairs, and should be considered in any such patient who presents with gastrointestinal bleeding. Blood loss is massive, as it gushes straight from the aorta into the intestine. Patients present with upper and lower GI haemorrhage and rapid collapse, and, if they are not taken to theatre urgently, mortality is almost inevitable.

5. B – Carcinoma of the stomach

This man presents with features of gastric cancer. Gastric cancer is the leading cause of cancer death worldwide. It is more common in Japanese populations, with a peak age range of 50–70 years. The five big medical risk factors for the development of gastric carcinoma are chronic peptic ulceration, *Helicobacter pylori* infection, gastric polyps, pernicious anaemia and Ménétrier disease. Pernicious anaemia is a condition characterized by vitamin B12 deficiency. In this condition, the body produces autoantibodies to parietal cells, which are the cells that release gastrin (a hormone that increases acid secretion). Because no gastrin is released in pernicious anaemia, there is reduced acid secretion and achlorhydria, which predisposes to gastric cancer. Ménétrier disease is a rare condition with hyperplasia of mucus-producing cells in the stomach. This results in a protein-losing enteropathy and reduced acid secretion. Carcinoma develops in 10% of cases of Ménétrier disease. Other risk factors for developing gastric cancer include blood group A, a family history, eating pickled foods, smoking and alcohol consumption.

Gastric cancer is usually an adenocarcinoma. Spread of this tumour is to lymph nodes, which can result in a Virchow node – supraclavicular lymphadenopathy on the left side as a result of internal malignancy. This is also known as Troisier sign. Gastric cancer can also spread to the ovaries via the peritoneum. The presence of an adenocarcinoma at the ovary that occurs secondary to gastric adenocarcinoma is known as a Krukenburg tumour. Gastric tumours may metastasize to the umbilicus. The presence of an umbilical metastasis is known as a Sister Joseph nodule. It looks like a hard, red lump adjacent to the umbilicus. The features of gastric carcinoma are often vague, and therefore such tumours often present late. Patients may present with epigastric pain that radiates to the back, vomiting due to pyloric obstruction, anorexia and weight loss. If liver metastases occur, jaundice may also be a feature. The diagnosis of gastric carcinoma is by endoscopy and biopsy. Management is by gastrectomy and lymph node clearance.

Adenocarcinoma is the most common form of oesophageal carcinoma and its incidence is rising. Most of these cancers have developed from Barrett's oesophagus, a condition that describes the metaplastic reaction from squamous to columnar cell types. High-grade dysplasia is treated with surgery in suitable candidates. A number of different approaches have been described, the principal ones being the Ivor Lewis, McKeown, and trans-hiatal.

Boerhaave syndrome is an eponymously named condition that describes oesophageal rupture secondary to vomiting. It results from a sudden increase in intra-oesophageal pressure combined with relatively low intra-thoracic pressure. The condition was described by the physician Herman Boerhaave after attending to a Dutch admiral who gorged on a feast and subsequently vomited. Symptoms include sudden-onset upper abdominal pain while vomiting. It is associated with a poor prognosis if untreated.

Rudolf Ludwig Virchow, German pathologist (1821–1902).
Charles Emile Troisier, French pathologist (1844–1919).
Sister Mary Joseph Dempsey, American nun and nurse (1856–1939).
Herman Boehaave, humanist and physician (1668–1738).

THEME 2: AIRWAY MANAGEMENT

1. C – Head tilt chin lift

This woman is drowsy after her operation and is not able to maintain her airway, as shown by the presence of stridor. Inspiratory grunting is a sign of upper airway obstruction. The *next* most appropriate step in her management is to open her airway, and this is best done by the head-tilt chin-lift manoeuvre: one hand is placed on the forehead to tilt the head back; the other hand is placed under the chin and lifted to help keep the mouth open. This posture is known as the 'sniffing the morning air' position. Another airway-opening manoeuvre, which can be used if the patient is unconscious, is the jaw thrust. This is done by placing two fingers under the angle of the mandible on both sides with the thumbs on the patient's chin and lifting the jaw upwards. The airway should also be examined for any obvious cause of obstruction, such as dentures, other foreign bodies or secretions.

2. G – Single-lumen cuffed endotracheal tube

This man will require a general anaesthetic, so a definitive airway is required. The endotracheal tube passes via the mouth into the trachea and allows for temporary mechanical ventilation of the patient. The cuffed end (a balloon) creates a seal to prevent aspiration of stomach contents.

3. B – Double-lumen cuffed endotracheal tube

The double-lumen endotracheal tube has been developed for lung and other intra-thoracic surgery. It allows for one lung to be ventilated while the other is collapsed to make surgery easier.

4. H – Single-lumen uncuffed endotracheal tube

This child, who has been involved in a fire, presents with respiratory distress and soot around his nasal passages. It is likely that he has suffered a smoke inhalation injury that requires endotracheal intubation. An uncuffed endotracheal tube is preferred in children, as the trachea is not as strong as in adults, and the use of a cuff increases the risk of tracheal damage with resulting stenosis. The risk of developing stenosis outweighs that of aspiration.

5. E – Needle cricothyroidotomy

This man needs urgent ventilation. Although an endotracheal tube would be ideal for short-term ventilation, attempts at this have failed and a surgical airway is required as soon as possible. Forming a percutaneous or surgical tracheostomy would be time-consuming and waste precious seconds, so an emergency needle cricothyroidotomy should be performed.

A needle cricothyroidotomy is performed by passing a wide-bore cannula through the skin and cricothyroid membrane, just below the thyroid cartilage (Adam's apple). This is a temporary measure and will allow for around 30 minutes of ventilation while a more permanent airway is made.

A bag and mask (also known as a bag valve mask) is a method of assisting ventilation should it be insufficient or absent. Care should be taken to ensure a tight seal between the mask and the patient's face. A nasopharyngeal airway is inserted along the floor of the nose to ensure the device enters the nasopharynx and not the frontal lobe having passed through the delicate cribiform plate! Lubricating jelly should be applied beforehand to ensure a smooth passage and minimize potential damage to the highly vascular turbinates. An oropharyngeal tube (commonly known as a Guedel airway) can be tolerated in patients with a GCS of 8 or less. In adults, it is positioned by inserting it into the oral cavity and inverting it 180 degrees so that its curvature parallels that of the base of the tongue. If a patient is able to tolerate such a device, their reduced level of consciousness is such that they are unable to protect their own airway and an anesthetist should be called urgently.

THEME 3: PANCREATIC TUMOURS

1. C – Insulinoma

Insulinomas are tumours of the pancreatic beta cells and are the most common of pancreatic endocrine tumours. Over-secretion of insulin leads to low glucose levels; hence the features of an insulinoma are similar to those of hypoglycaemia. Patients may complain of being weak, sweaty, confused and hungry and having diarrhoea. The diagnosis of insulinoma may be helped by eliciting Whipple's triad of symptoms: attacks are induced by starvation, there is hypoglycaemia during attacks, and the symptoms are relieved by eating. Insulinomas must be distinguished from inappropriate insulin administration – this is done by measuring insulin and C-peptide levels in the blood. C-peptide is a product from the cleavage of the insulin precursor, proinsulin. In cases of insulinoma, both C-peptide and insulin will be raised, as there is endogenous insulin production. In people who are administering excess insulin, the insulin levels but not the C-peptide levels will be raised. Most cases of insulinoma are benign (80%), but, because of the malignant potential, management is by excision.

Allen Oldfather Whipple, American surgeon (1881–1963).

2. F – VIPoma

A VIPoma is a tumour of the pancreatic islets that secrete vasoactive intestinal polypeptide (VIP). VIP is a peptide hormone that stimulates the secretion of water and electrolytes in the intestines. Because of these actions, a VIPoma presents with severe, watery diarrhoea, dehydration and hypokalaemia. VIP also inhibits stomach acid secretion, so there is no gastric acid output (known as achlorhydria). Other features are hyperglycaemia and hypercalcaemia. Plasma VIP levels are raised. The treatment of VIPomas is by excision, but symptoms can also be improved by the drug octreotide, a synthetic analogue of somatostatin that inhibits VIP.

3. B – Glucagonoma

Glucagon is secreted by the alpha cells of the pancreatic islets. Its function results in increased blood glucose, so it does the opposite job to insulin. The excess glucagon production that occurs with glucagonomas, and the subsequent glucagon/insulin imbalance, results in diabetes mellitus. Eighty percent of glucagonomas also present with necrolytic migratory erythema, a blistering rash that occurs around the buttocks, groins and legs, and eventually crusts over, leaving a brown scar. This neuroendocrine tumour is rare with just 1 per million people being diagnosed with it each year. It is also associated with the MEN 1 syndrome.

4. A – Gastrinoma

Usually in peptic ulcer disease, ulcerations are found in the stomach and proximal duodenum. This man presents with peptic ulcer disease and has multiple, larger ulcers in his duodenum and jejunum – this presentation is typical of a gastrinoma.

A gastrinoma is a tumour of the G cells of the pancreas that results in an increased secretion of the hormone gastrin. Gastrin stimulates the production of gastric acid, so a tumour that produces large amounts of gastrin will result in a high acid output in the stomach. This predisposes to the formation of multiple, large peptic ulcers in unusual anatomical positions, along with their complications, such as bleeding and perforation. The overproduction of acid will also result in diarrhoea.

The features that result from a gastrin-secreting tumour are known as Zollinger-Ellison syndrome. The diagnosis of a gastrinoma is made by elevated serum gastrin levels. The tumour itself may be visualized by CT or MRI. Treatment is by excision or with proton pump inhibitors to inhibit acid secretion.

Robert Milton Zollinger, American surgeon (1903–1992).

Edwin Homer Ellison, American surgeon (1918–1970).

5. E – Somatostatinoma

Somatostatin is secreted by the delta cells of the pancreas. Its functions are twofold: to inhibit the release of glucagon and insulin, and to suppress the exocrine secretion of pancreatic enzymes. Somatostatinomas, which produce large amounts of somatostatin, therefore have predictable features. Because insulin and glucagon secretion is suppressed, patients have diabetes. Secondly, because there is suppression of the exocrine pancreas, there is malabsorption and steatorrhoea. Another feature of somatostatinomas is gallstone disease as somatostatin suppresses gall bladder contraction. Management is by excision, but somatostatinomas are often aggressively malignant and have a poor prognosis.

THEME 4: ENDOCRINE DISORDERS

1. A – Acromegaly

Acromegaly is caused by a growth hormone (GH)-secreting tumour of the anterior pituitary gland. The functions of GH include lipolysis, protein synthesis and gluconeogenesis – in other words, it is an anabolic hormone. Patients with acromegaly may present with headaches, excessive sweating, thick/oily skin, hypertrophy of soft tissues (large nose/lips/tongue and 'spade-like' hands), large viscera, prognathism (protruding lower jaw) and prominent supraorbital ridges. Other associations are carpal tunnel syndrome, diabetes and hypertension. The pituitary mass may result in features of a space-occupying lesion in the brain, i.e. an early morning headache that is worse on coughing and straining. If a GH-secreting tumour occurs in children before the bone epiphyses have fused, the long bones grow rapidly and gigantism results.

Acromegaly from Greek *akros* = extremities + *megas* = large.

It is important to treat acromegaly, because it is associated with an increased risk of atheromatous disease and colon cancer. The diagnosis is made by measuring GH levels before and after a 75 g glucose load (an oral glucose tolerance test).

Glucose normally suppresses GH secretion, but in acromegaly, the glucose load has little effect. Surgical treatment is by trans-sphenoid surgery. Medical therapy is with somatostatin analogues (e.g. intramuscular octreotide), which inhibit GH secretion.

2. L – Nelson syndrome

This woman has been treated for Cushing disease in the past. Cushing disease is the presence of an ACTH-secreting tumour in the pituitary that results in excess cortisol and features of Cushing syndrome. The treatment of Cushing disease is usually by removal of the primary tumour. However, in occasional cases where the tumour is occult, bilateral adrenalectomy is performed to eliminate the production of cortisol. The lack of cortisol's negative feedback on the pituitary allows the pre-existing pituitary ACTH tumour to grow rapidly. This process is known as Nelson syndrome and occurs after 20% of bilateral adrenalectomies. Melanocyte-stimulating hormone (MSH) is created as a by-product of the cleavage of proopiomelanocortin (POMC), the precursor to ACTH. It is this MSH that results in the hyperpigmentation seen in Nelson syndrome.

Nelson D, Meakin J, Thorn G. ACTH-producing pituitary tumors following adrenalectomy for Cushing's syndrome. *Ann Intern Med* 1960; 52: 560–9.

3. I – Multiple endocrine neoplasia type 1

This young patient has multiple peptic ulcers that are suggestive of a gastrinoma, a pancreatic tumour. The brain tumour that causes lactation is a prolactinoma, a tumour of the pituitary gland. The combination of pancreatic endocrine tumours with a prolactinoma suggests multiple endocrine neoplasia (MEN) type 1.

There are three types of MEN, all of which are autosomal dominant conditions. MEN type 1 (Wermer syndrome) includes the presence of parathyroid adenomas, pancreatic islet-cell tumours and pituitary adenomas. MEN type 2 (Sipple syndrome; previously termed MEN type 2a) comprises parathyroid adenomas, medullary carcinoma of the thyroid and phaeochromocytoma. Finally, MEN type 3 (previously termed MEN type 2b) includes the presence of the tumours of MEN type 2 but with the addition of multiple mucosal neuromas of the gastrointestinal tract and a marfanoid phenotype.

Paul Wermer, American physician (1898–1975).

John Sipple, American physician (b1930).

4. E – Conn syndrome

This woman presents with polyuria, polydipsia and muscle cramps associated with a high sodium and low potassium. This suggests a diagnosis of Conn syndrome.

Conn syndrome results from an aldosterone-secreting adenoma of the adrenal gland. Aldosterone causes sodium reabsorption and potassium excretion in the kidneys. Excess aldosterone results in sodium and water retention, leading to high blood pressure and oedema. Surplus potassium excretion results in hypokalaemia, the features of which include muscle cramps and weakness, polyuria (secondary to renal tubular damage, i.e. nephrogenic diabetes insipidus), and polydipsia. The diagnosis of Conn syndrome can be made by measuring serum aldosterone and renin levels – aldosterone will be raised and renin levels will be reduced due to negative feedback. Many antihypertensive medications interfere with these hormones, so it is important to stop these for at least 6 weeks prior to testing. Initial management is with spironolactone, an aldosterone antagonist. Once the adenoma has been localized (using CT), it can be surgically removed.

Jerome Conn, American endocrinologist (1907–1981).

5. K – Multiple endocrine neoplasia type 3

This patient is likely to have MEN type 3 (previously termed MEN type 2b), an autosomal dominant condition characterized by phaeochromocytoma, parathyroid adenomas, medullary thyroid cancer, multiple mucosal neuromas and a marfanoid habitus (e.g. tall stature, arachnodactyly, high-arched palate).

Addison disease is a condition that describes adrenal insufficiency. The most common cause worldwide is tuberculosis, but it is most commonly autoimmune in origin in the UK. In severe cases, Addison disease can develop into an Addisonian crisis where severe hypotension and coma are seen. Waterhouse Friderichsen syndrome is characterized by bleeding into the adrenal glands as a result of *Neisseria meningitidis* infection. Carcinoid tumours are apudomas (endocrine tumours that arise from APUD cells) that arise from enterochromaffin cells. The appendix is the most common site. Patients present with symptoms associated with 5HT (serotonin) excess, namely flushing, diarrhea and colicky abdominal pain. Congenital adrenal hyperplasia is a term used to encompass several conditions that relate to enzyme insufficiency of the adrenal glands. It results in deficiencies of corticosteroids, mineralocorticoids and/or sex steroids.

Antoine Marfan, French paediatrician (1858–1942).

THEME 5: MANAGEMENT OF ABDOMINAL PAIN

1. C – Cefuroxime and metronidazole

Diverticulitis results from inflammation of colonic diverticulae. A diverticulum, defined as an abnormal outpouching of a hollow viscus into surrounding tissue, may be 'true' i.e. involving all layers of the viscus wall (such as a Meckel diverticulum) or 'false' (as in a colonic diverticulum) where only some of layers (usually the inner layers) protrude outwards.

Diverticulitis often occurs due to faeces becoming lodged and stagnant within a diverticulum. Acute diverticulitis presents with central abdominal pain that eventually localizes to the left iliac fossa, with vomiting, diarrhoea, fever, local guarding and a leukocytosis. There is a risk that an inflamed diverticulum can perforate – either into the peritoneal cavity, resulting in peritonitis, or into adjacent structures such as the bladder, resulting in a fistula. Diverticulitis is the most common cause of a colovescical fistula, which presents with the passage of bubbles in the urine (pneumaturia). Other presentations of diverticulitis include rectal bleeding, paracolic abscesses and stricture +/– obstruction. The best way to demonstrate the presence of diverticula, especially in the acute phase of diverticulitis, is with a CT scan. Treatment is with fluids and appropriate antibiotics, such as cefuroxime and metronidazole. If conservative therapy fails, surgery is indicated. Usually this takes the form of a Hartmann procedure where the rectosigmoid is resected leaving the patient with a temporary end colostomy or ileostomy which can be reversed once the sepsis has resolved.

2. E – Metoclopramide

Gastric stasis, or gastroparesis, is characterized by an inefficient, incomplete emptying of the stomach, resulting in early satiety, bloating, anorexia, weight loss and vomiting. It is usually associated with problems of the vagus nerve. People with diabetes, some neurological disorders and scleroderma are prone to developing gastroparesis. Anticholinergic drugs and gastric operations are also risk factors. The diagnosis of gastroparesis is confirmed by a gastric emptying test: the patient is asked to eat a radiolabelled scrambled egg (or something similar!) and serial X-rays are taken of the gastrointestinal tract over a few days. Management is initially with prokinetic drugs, including metoclopramide, erythromycin and domperidone. If these measures fail, a gastric pacing device may improve symptoms. Both metoclopramide and domperidone are dopamine receptor antagonists and act to increase small bowel transit, gastric emptying and increase lower oesophageal sphincter tone.

3. G – Omeprazole, clarithromycin and metronidazole

This man has proven peptic ulceration on endoscopy. Peptic ulcers are most commonly caused by non-steroidal anti-inflammatory drugs and *Helicobacter pylori* infection. *Helicobacter pylori* is a Gram-negative, spiral-shaped rod that can colonize gastric-type mucosa, whether that is in the stomach itself or gastric-type metaplasia in the oesophagus or duodenum. *H. pylori* infection is found in 50% of the over-50s, but most people with it are asymptomatic. *H. pylori* produces urease, an enzyme that converts urea into ammonia. The ammonia it releases neutralizes the acidic pH around it; hence this bacterium can live in the harsh acidic environment of the stomach. *H. pylori* damages gastric mucosa by releasing toxic ammonia and cytokines as well as by increasing stomach acid secretion by stimulating gastrin production.

Peptic ulcer disease presents with intermittent epigastric pain that radiates to the back. The pain may start immediately after eating, but it usually starts 2 hours after eating. Because the pain often starts so long after eating, patients commonly think that it is brought about by *not* eating – hence they complain of so-called 'hunger pain'. In reality, you cannot tell if an ulcer is gastric or duodenal based on the time relationship between eating and the onset of pain. The pain of peptic ulcers tends to be worse with spicy foods, but is relieved by milk and alkalis.

The best investigation for peptic ulcers is an upper GI endoscopy, or OGD. It is important during endoscopy to take multiple biopsies of the edge and centre of ulcers to exclude any malignant transformation within these lesions. One of the biopsies is tested for *H. pylori* using the CLO test (the '*Campylobacter*-like organism' test – so-called since when the bacteria was first discovered, its morphology was seen to be similar, but not identical, to that of *Campylobacter*). In this test, some urea is placed on the biopsy and pH paper is left on top. If *H. pylori* is present, it will produce ammonia and increase the pH of the medium. If *H. pylori* is found in conjunction with peptic ulceration, eradication therapy is instituted. This consists of a 7-day course of a proton pump inhibitor (PPI) with clarithromycin and metronidazole. This is known as triple therapy. Following the course, the PPI alone is continued and a repeat endoscopy performed after 6–8 weeks.

4. F – Ofloxacin and metronidazole
This woman is presenting with pelvic inflammatory disease (PID), which is most commonly caused by *Chlamydia trachomatis* and *Neisseria gonorrhoea*. Ofloxacin and metronidazole is a typical regimen for PID, covering the main two causes as well as anaerobes and parasitic infections.

5. I – Steroids
This woman presents with an exacerbation of her ulcerative colitis. This should be managed with steroids, orally or rectally.

Ulcerative colitis (UC) is an inflammatory condition of the rectum that extends for a variable distance proximally along the colon without skip lesions. It is most common in females and tends to present in early adulthood with crampy abdominal pains, bloody diarrhoea, fever, anorexia and weight loss. In severe attacks, the colon can dilate massively (>6 cm) with a high risk of perforation – this is known as toxic megacolon. The pathology of UC includes bowel mucosal oedema with contact bleeding and shallow irregular ulcers. The diagnosis of UC is confirmed by sigmoidoscopy and biopsy. A barium enema will demonstrate a smooth, narrow, featureless bowel with loss of haustrations (the 'lead-pipe' colon).

UC is associated with many extra-intestinal manifestations, including erythema nodosum, pyoderma gangrenosum and sclerosing cholangitis. Erythema nodosum describes the presence of purple palpable lesions that usually occur on the shins. These lesions are painful to touch and are managed simply with NSAIDs. Pyoderma gangrenosum describes the appearance of necrotic, deep, well-defined ulcers with a bluish edge and tend to occur on the legs.

UC is managed medically in the first instance. Steroids, given systemically or rectally, help induce remission in acute attacks. Disease-modifying drugs, e.g. azathioprine and mesalazine, can be taken regularly to reduce the frequency and severity of remissions. People with UC are encouraged to eat a high-protein diet and have vitamin supplements. Fulminating disease is defined as the passage of 6 or more bloody motions per day, with fever, tachycardia and hypoalbuminaemia. Fulminating disease is an indication for surgical intervention. UC is associated with an increased risk of developing colorectal carcinomas. For this reason, regular colonoscopy is advised. Some people choose instead to have a prophylactic total colectomy with either a permanent ileostomy or ileo-anal anastomosis. The risk of malignant transformation equates to roughly 1% per year. If an ileo-anal anastomosis is formed, surveillance is still required.

THEME 6: SKIN LESIONS

1. F – Kaposi sarcoma
Kaposi sarcoma is a malignant tumour of vascular endothelium that gives rise to plaques and nodules in the skin and mucous membranes that have a bruise-like appearance. It is associated with underlying human

herpes virus 8 (HHV-8) infection in people who are immunosuppressed (such as those with AIDS or patients on immunosuppressants following organ transplantation). Before the advent of AIDS, Kaposi sarcoma was a rare sporadic tumour that occurred in male Italians and Ashkenazi Jews. Biopsy of the lesions is required to confirm diagnosis, and symptomatic treatment is with radiotherapy.

Moriz Kohn Kaposi, Hungarian dermatologist (1837–1902).

2. D – Granuloma annulare

Granuloma annulare is a condition characterized by small reddish papules that are arranged in a ring. It usually occurs on the backs of the hands or feet and is often associated with diabetes mellitus. Granuloma annulare is usually asymptomatic and lesions fade after a year. Although its aetiology is unknown, it is thought to be due to a T-cell-mediated reaction.

Annulare, from Latin *anus* = ring.

3. I – Pyogenic granuloma

A pyogenic granuloma is an acquired haemangioma (localized excess of proliferating capillaries). Lesions most often occur on the head, trunk, hands and feet and characteristically have a tendency to bleed heavily on minimal trauma and enlarge rapidly over 2–3 weeks. They develop at a site of trauma (e.g. a thorn prick) as a bright red nodule, although hyperkeratosis of the underlying healthy epidermis can give them a white appearance. Note that they are neither pyogenic nor a granuloma. It affects the young and old extremes of age, but is most common in pregnant women. These lesions are benign and are managed by excision, although smaller lesions may resolve spontaneously.

4. H – Neurofibroma

Neurofibromas are benign neoplasms of the nerve sheaths of central or peripheral nerves that feel firm and rubbery. Neurofibromas may be single or multiple, as in neurofibromatosis. Neurofibromatosis (NF) is an autosomal dominant disorder characterized by multiple neurofibromas, coffee-coloured macules (café-au-lait patches) and axillary freckling, with a risk of developing central nervous system tumours (acoustic neuroma, optic glioma and meningioma), iris fibromas (Lisch nodules) and phaeochromocytomas. There are two types of NF: NF1 (von Recklinghausen disease) is the 'peripheral' form that displays the cutaneous manifestations; and NF2 is the 'central' form, with bilateral central nervous systems tumours and very few cutaneous features.

Friedrich von Recklinghausen, German pathologist (1833–1910).

5. A – Cellulitis

The features of erythema, swelling, local pain and blistering of an area of skin in the pyrexial, unwell patient suggest a diagnosis of cellulitis. Cellulitis is an infection of the subcutaneous tissues that is most commonly caused by *Streptococcus pyogenes*. Treatment is by broad-spectrum IV antibiotics, such as flucloxacillin and benzylpenicillin.

THEME 7: CONDITIONS OF THE NOSE

1. G – Foreign body

A foreign body in the nostril can result in chronic inflammation, presenting with a foul-smelling, blood-stained purulent discharge. Young children commonly insert objects into their nose and, after recovering from the initial trauma, forget that they are there! Treatment is by urgent removal of the object, which may have to be done under a general anaesthetic. There is a risk that foreign bodies in the nose can be inhaled.

2. K – Spontaneous epistaxis

There are many causes of epistaxis. These include foreign bodies, chemical irritation, intranasal tumours, surgery, and bleeding diatheses. The most common cause of recurrent epistaxis in children is nose-picking. In this case, there is trauma to the mucosal lining of the nose. Bleeding from the nose most commonly occurs from Little's area, a particularly vascular region at the anterior septum that is supplied by the anterior ethmoidal artery, superior labial artery and the sphenopalatine artery (branches of the internal and external carotids). To treat a small bleed from Little's area apply digital pressure on the lower nose (to compress the vessels), while leaning the head forward (to prevent aspiration of blood). If this does not work, the mucosa can be cauterized using a silver nitrate stick, or nasal packing can be instituted.

Epistaxis, from Greek *epi* = from + *stactic* = drip; 'dripping from', especially with regard to blood from the nose.

It is still debated as to whether or not epistaxis is associated with hypertension, as both are frequent in the general population. Some hypothesize that epistaxis occurs as a result of end-organ damage that is associated with long-standing hypertension.

3. C – Acute maxillary sinusitis

Acute sinusitis is inflammation of the paranasal sinuses that usually occurs following a bacterial upper respiratory tract infection. The pain of acute sinusitis is worse on bending and coughing. The site of the pain depends on which sinus is affected. Acute maxillary sinusitis causes pain over the cheek, which may be referred to the teeth. Acute frontal sinusitis causes pain above the eyes. Acute ethmoid and sphenoid sinusitis can result in pain between or behind the eyes. In reality, however, the site of sinusitis may be very difficult to distinguish. In maxillary sinusitis, a skull X-ray may show a fluid level on the affected side. Treatment is with antibiotics (amoxicillin) and analgesia. Vasoconstricting nose drops (1% ephedrine) aid drainage of the sinus. Sinusitis can be acute (<4 weeks), subacute (4–12 weeks) or chronic (>12 weeks). The evolution of man, adapting to stand on two legs instead of four, has caused a problem with the drainage of the maxillary sinus. Now the outflow to the sinus is sited superiorly, and is no longer assisted by gravity. Consequently, it is the maxillary sinus that is most commonly affected.

4. E – Chemical irritation

It is likely that this man has chemical irritation of the nasal mucosa secondary to cocaine use. Cocaine is a potent vasoconstrictor, and chronic use can result in ischaemic necrosis of the nasal septum, eventually leading to a septal defect. Similarly, due to its action on the coronary vasculature, cocaine use should be considered as a potential cause of myocardial infarction in young 'fit' individuals (in fact, it is the most common cause of myocardial infarction in this age group).

Another possible cause for this man's symptoms could be Wegener granulomatosis. Wegener granulomatosis is an autoimmune vasculitis characterized by recurrent epistaxis, haemoptysis and renal disease. Wegener's can result in perforation of the nasal septum, resulting in a saddle-nose deformity. It is associated with cytoplasmic anti-neutrophil cytoplasmic antibodies (cANCA). This is unlikely to be the correct answer to this scenario, as this man has no other symptoms.

Friedrich Wegener, German pathologist (1907–1990).

5. D – Allergic rhinitis

The features of allergic rhinitis (runny nose, sneezing, conjunctival irritation) occur when exposure to certain allergens results in IgE-mediated mast cell degranulation. This causes vasodilation and increased capillary permeability. Allergic rhinitis can be seasonal (e.g. to pollen) or perennial (e.g. to house dust mite, animal dander). It is associated with atopy – a hereditary disorder of susceptibility to IgE-mediated reactions, including asthma and infantile eczema. Management of allergic rhinitis is by avoiding allergens, antihistamines and topical steroids (beclometasone nasal spray). Even though this man only developed these features at age 23, allergic rhinitis is still the most likely diagnosis.

Non-allergic rhinitis presents similarly to allergic rhinitis, but there is no type I hypersensitivity reaction. Instead, there is an association with eosinophilia. Patients suffer symptoms all year round and can develop nasal polyps. Nasal polyps cause nasal obstruction and discharge, and are usually bilateral. Polyps can shrink with steroid use, but definitive treatment is by polypectomy under anaesthetic (local or general).

THEME 8: PAEDIATRIC ORTHOPAEDIC CONDITIONS

1. F – Slipped upper femoral epiphysis

Slipped upper femoral epiphysis describes posterolateral displacement of the femoral head, following a fracture through the physis (growth plate). Progressive displacement occurs, leading to external rotation of the hip and shortening of the lower limb. It occurs most common in boys aged 10–15 years during their adolescent growth spurt and is associated with obesity, microgenitalia, hypothyroidism, familial history and a tall stature. Twenty percent of cases are bilateral. Slipped upper femoral epiphysis presents with a limp and hip pain referred to the knee. It may follow minor trauma. There may be restriction in abduction and internal rotation of the hip. When flexed, the hip tends to move into an externally rotated position. The diagnosis is confirmed on a lateral-view X-ray of the affected hip. Management is by surgical pinning of the epiphysis. In severe slips, open reduction or corrective osteotomies may be required. Complications of a slipped upper femoral epiphysis include premature epiphyseal fusion, avascular necrosis and early-onset arthritis.

2. D – Perthes disease

Perthes disease (or Legg–Clave–Perthes disease) is a degenerative disease of the hip. There is ischaemia of the femoral head involving the epiphysis and adjacent metaphysis (resulting in avascular necrosis). A period of fragmentation and progressive deformity of the hip is followed by revascularization and re-ossification over 2–3 years. Perthes disease is five times more common in boys and usually occurs between 5 and 10 years of age. It presents with insidious-onset hip pain (which may be referred to the knee) and a limp. It is bilateral in 10% of cases. Diagnosis is by lateral X-ray of the affected hip, which shows an increased density and reduced size of the femoral head. The femoral head later becomes fragmented and irregular.

Management in mild disease is by bed rest and traction. In more severe cases, the femoral head needs to be 'covered' by the acetabulum so that it can act as a mould for the re-ossifying epiphysis. This is achieved by maintaining the hip in abduction (by placing the child in Gallows traction) or by surgical femoral osteotomy. The prognosis of Perthes disease is usually good. However, if the child is under 6 years, or if more than half the epiphysis is involved, there is an increased risk of deformity of the femoral head, with subsequent degenerative osteoarthritis in adult life.

Georg Clemens Perthes, German surgeon (1869–1927).

3. J – Transient synovitis

Transient synovitis (irritable hip) is the most common cause of acute hip pain in prepubescent children and often follows a viral infection. Features include sudden-onset hip pain that radiates to the knee, a slight limp and a reduced range of movement, especially external rotation. There is no pain at rest and minimal systemic symptoms. Investigations, such as full blood count, acute-phase proteins, joint X-ray and blood cultures, are negative. Ultrasound investigation may demonstrate a small effusion. Management is with analgesia, bed rest and skin traction. Irritable hip usually resolves in 7–10 days.

4. A – Developmental dysplasia of the hip

Developmental dysplasia of the hip (DDH, or congenital dislocation of the hip) is a spectrum of disorders ranging from partial subluxation to frank dislocation of the hip. It is thought that high concentrations of the maternal hormone relaxin contribute to the laxity of the hip joint. DDH is found in 1 in 1000 births, and it is six times more common in females. The left hip is more likely to be dislocated than the right. Risk factors for DDH include a positive family history, breech delivery, spinal/neuromuscular abnormalities (e.g. spina bifida, talipes equinovarus) and oligohydramnios.

Neonatal screening for DDH is by two methods: Barlow's test (the hip can easily be displaced posteriorly out of the acetabulum on adduction of the leg with posterior pressure) and Ortolani manoeuvre (the femoral head can be reduced back into the acetabulum on abduction of the leg with anterior pressure). These tests are routinely done at birth and 6 weeks of age. DDH may present with asymmetric skin folds, limited abduction, shortening of the affected limb and limp. If spotted early, DDH responds to conservative treatment. The hips can be placed in abduction (using a Craig splint) or the child can be put in a restraining device (Pavlik harness) for several months. Progress should be monitored by ultrasound or X-ray. If conservative measures fail, open reduction and femoral osteotomy may be required. Necrosis of the femoral head is a potential complication of DDH. If left untreated, patients develop a severe limp, limb shortening and early-onset osteoarthritis.

Marino Ortolani, Italian paediatrician (1904–1983).

Sir Thomas Barlow, English physician and paediatrician (1845–1945).

5. H – Still's disease

Still's disease is a systemic form of juvenile arthritis that is thought to be an autoimmune disorder. It usually begins at the age of 3–4 years and is more common in girls. Features of Still's disease include intermittent high pyrexia and a salmon-pink rash with aches and pains of the joints and muscles. Other features are hepatosplenomegaly, lymphadenopathy and pericarditis. Inflammatory markers such as C-reactive protein will be raised; however antinuclear antibodies (ANA) and rheumatoid factor are usually negative. Management options include physiotherapy, resting splints, NSAIDs, disease-modifying drugs (e.g. methotrexate and ciclosporin) and steroids. The younger the age of onset of Still's disease, the worse is the prognosis.

Sir George Frederick Still, English physician (1861–1941).

THEME 9: MANAGEMENT OF PROSTATE DISEASE

Prostate cancer is predominantly a disease of older men, although 20% of cases occur below the age of 65. Management of the disease is dependent upon the patient's wishes, life expectancy and disease progression (staging).

Staging of prostate cancer is with the TNM (tumour, node, metastases) system. Tumour staging:

T1 Clinically unapparent tumour not palpable or visible by imaging
T2 Tumour confined to prostate, palpable or visible on imaging
T3 Tumour extends through prostatic capsule, with or without seminal vesicle involvement
T4 Tumour fixed or invading adjacent structures other than the seminal vesicles
N1 Is used to denote lymph node involvement
M1 Represents the presence of distant metastases

The most common site of prostatic metastases is the bone (osteosclerotic lesions), which can result in bone pain and pathological fractures. T1 or T2 disease is considered to be localized and potentially curable. If curative treatment is considered, an MRI scan is initially required to stage the tumour.

1. A – Active surveillance

This man has been diagnosed with localized disease only. He is now 87 and therefore will not have much life expectancy. Patients with localized asymptomatic tumours (T1–T2) who have a life expectancy less than 10 years can be managed with active surveillance, as it is unlikely that the localized prostate malignancy will drastically affect their morbidity. Active surveillance is with regular PSA measurements and digital rectal examinations, and at least one repeat core biopsy. It is also the preferred option for low-risk men who are candidates for radical treatment. In patients who have a life expectancy >10 years with localized prostate cancer, potentially curative therapy in the form of a radical prostatectomy or radiotherapy are valid options, as there is a higher risk of progression of disease in the patient's lifetime.

2. D – External-beam radiotherapy

This man is experiencing symptoms from bony metastases of prostate cancer. He is currently taking hormonal therapy. The aim of hormonal therapy is to prevent the testosterone-induced progression of prostate cancer and reduce the risk of complications such as pathological fractures and spinal cord compression. Although initial response is good, prostate tumours eventually become androgen-independent, rendering hormonal therapies useless. Symptomatic bone metastases may then be improved by a course of external-beam radiotherapy to the affected area. If radiotherapy and analgesics fail to relieve symptoms, strontium-89 and bisphosphonates should be commenced.

3. B – Brachytherapy

Radical prostatectomy involves removal of the prostate with re-anastomosis of the bladder neck to the urethra, with or without pelvic lymph node dissection. It carries a 70% risk of erectile dysfunction and a 5% risk of incontinence.

Brachytherapy has two forms. The first involves the implantation of radioactive 'seeds' into the prostate gland. The second, known as temporary brachytherapy, involves the insertion of thin tubes through the perineal skin (usually under GA) into the prostate. A computer is used to control how long a radioactive source flows through these tubes. The ionizing radiation damages DNA and increases apoptosis.

Brachytherapy is a popular method of treating localized prostate disease, as there is a lower rate of complications (30% impotence, 1% incontinence). It can be performed on an outpatient basis, and there is a similar long-term outcome when compared to those who undergo radical prostatectomy. Side effects of the radiation include radiation proctitis.

4. E – Finasteride

This man has benign prostatic hyperplasia (BPH) with symptoms that are troubling him. Patients with mild, untroubling symptoms can be managed conservatively by active surveillance. For those with worse symptoms, medical management is recommended. The two drug groups used to manage BPH are the adrenergic antagonists (e.g. doxazosin and alfuzosin) and the 5α-reductase inhibitors (e.g. finasteride). The adrenergic antagonists act on α_1 receptors on the prostate and bladder neck smooth muscle to reduce smooth muscle tone and reduce bladder outflow resistance. Their main side effect is postural hypotension. The 5α-reductase inhibitors block the action of 5α-reductase, which converts testosterone to dihydrotestosterone (the active form, which encourages prostate hyperplasia). They are effective on men with large prostates (>40 g), but these drugs can take months to have an effect. Overall, adrenergic antagonists are the first-line medical management for BPH, except for men with large prostates (>40 g) or raised PSA levels, in whom 5α-reductase inhibitors are the initial therapy of choice.

5. G – Transurethral resection of prostate

Surgery is indicated for patients who have inadequate symptomatic relief with medical therapy. It is also required in men who have bladder stones, recurrent infections or present with acute urinary retention. Operative management is by transurethral resection of the prostate (TURP) unless the prostate is very large (>90 g), in which case open prostatectomy may be required.

THEME 10: STATISTICS

1. E – 75%

The sensitivity of an investigation is its ability to detect a truly positive result. It is calculated as follows:

Sensitivity = number of true positives/(number of true positives + number of false negatives) × 100

Sensitivity = 150/(150 + 50) × 100 = 75%

2. F – 83%

The specificity is the ability of an investigation to detect a truly negative test result.

Specificity = number of true negatives/(number of true negatives + number of false positives) × 100

Specificity = 250/(250 + 50) × 100 = 5/6 × 100 ≈ 83%

3. E – 75%

The positive predictive value (PPV) describes the probability that a condition can be confirmed given a positive test result.

PPV = (number of true positives/total number of positives) × 100

PPV = (150/200) × 100 = 3/4 × 100 = 75%

4. F – 83%

The negative predictive value (NPV) describes the probability that a condition can be ruled out given a negative test result.

NPV = (number of true negatives/total number of negatives) × 100

NPV = (250/300) × 100 = 5/6 × 100 ≈ 83%

5. J – 4.5

The likelihood ratio is the likelihood that a given test result will be positive in a patient with a certain disorder compared with the likelihood that a positive result would be expected in a patient without that disorder.

Likelihood ratio = sensitivity/(1 – specificity)

Likelihood ratio = 0.75/(1 – 5/6) = 4.5

THEME 11: KNEE INJURIES

1. H – Patellar fracture

This man has sustained a direct blow to his patella that would have resulted in a fracture. The patella can be fractured either by a sudden, violent contraction of the quadriceps muscle or by a direct blow. The resulting pain is severe and localized, and there is usually a haemarthrosis (blood in the joint).

Patients will be unable to extend the knee due to disruption of the extensor mechanism of the leg. The inability to straight leg raise is not a specific test for patella fractures, but is a sensitive test of the extensor mechanism.

2. A – Anterior cruciate injury

The knee contains two cruciate ligaments: the anterior cruciate ligament (ACL), which prevents forward displacement of the tibia relative to the femur; and the posterior cruciate ligament (PCL), which inhibits backward displacement. ACL injury typically results from rotational stress on the fixed weight-bearing joint. When a cruciate ligament becomes damaged, the patient will feel or hear a 'pop' and there will be immediate haemarthrosis of the joint. This is unlike meniscal tears, where the effusion takes some time to develop.

Latin, *crux* = cross; the ligaments cross each other.

Cruciate ligament injuries can be determined easily on clinical examination. If the ACL is damaged then the tibia can be drawn forward excessively when the knee is flexed to 90° (the anterior drawer test). Lachman test is a variation of this, where the tibia can be pulled forwards markedly with the knee flexed at 20°. In PCL injuries, the tibia can be pushed backwards excessively by a force placed just below the patella (the posterior drawer test). When examining for an ACL injury, look for posterior sag. This should be done first as a disrupted PCL may be mistaken for a falsely positive anterior drawer test as the tibia may be drawn forwards to a neutral position. Posterior sag is best examined for by putting the patient's ankles together with knees flexed to 45° and looking from the side to see if both legs are parallel.

3. K – Tibial plateau fracture

A strong valgus force, such as that transmitted by the bumper of a moving car, may result in a fracture of the lateral tibial plateau. Most tibial plateau fractures can be diagnosed by conventional radiography although a CT scan is usually required for operative planning. Classification uses the Schatzker system.

4. E – Medial meniscus tear

Injuries of the menisci are common in men under 45 years. Tears are usually caused by a twisting force when the knee is in flexion, and medial meniscal injuries are more common than lateral ones. The menisci are mainly avascular, so injuries to these cartilages result in the development of a synovial fluid effusion over the course of a few hours. This is in contrast to cruciate ligament injuries, which are accompanied by the immediate (within minutes) development of a haemarthrosis. To develop a sudden haemarthrosis, something must bleed within the knee capsule itself, therefore only intra-capsular ligament injures or fractures can cause this. Rupture to the collateral ligaments (extra-capsular) or meniscal tears will not cause a haemarthrosis by themselves.

Patients who damage a meniscus complain of knee pain with an inability to straighten the knee. Some patients may also experience intermittent locking of the knee. An effusion occurs hours later and lasts around 2 weeks. On examination, there will be tenderness either along the medial or lateral joint line (depending on whether the medial or lateral meniscus is damaged).

5. D – Medial collateral injury

This man has suffered a valgus (outward) force on his right leg. A large valgus force upon the knee will result in damage to the medial collateral ligament, whereas a significant varus (inward) force will cause lateral collateral ligament damage. Features include pain and instability of the knee. On examination, there will be tenderness over the area of the damaged ligament. Considerable laxity is seen when a valgus force is placed on the leg (for medial ligament injuries).

In cases of severe valgus force upon the knee, a combination of medial collateral ligament, medial meniscus and anterior cruciate ligament injuries can occur. This is known as O'Donoghue's terrible triad.

THEME 12: MANAGEMENT OF ANORECTAL CONDITIONS

1. E – Injection sclerotherapy

Haemorrhoids result from dilatation of the superior rectal arteries within the anal canal. Risk factors for their development include chronic constipation, pregnancy and portal hypertension. Haemorrhoids are graded as follows: first-degree haemorrhoids are confined to the anal canal; second-degree prolapse on defaecation and reduce spontaneously; and third-degree prolapse on defaecation and require manual replacement. Presenting features of haemorrhoids include fresh rectal bleeding following defaecation, which is noticed on the paper when wiping. Other features are itching, a dragging sensation and mucus discharge. The diagnosis of haemorrhoids is made by per rectum examination or proctoscopy. The haemorrhoids are found at the 3, 7 and 11 o'clock positions when the patient is in the lithotomy position.

Haemorrhoids, from Greek *haima* = blood + *rhoia* = to flow; 'likely to bleed'; also known as piles from Latin *pila* = balls.

Asymptomatic haemorrhoids should be managed only with conservative measures, such as increasing dietary fibre and water. Injection sclerotherapy may be used for symptomatic first- and second-degree haemorrhoids. This involves the injection of phenol into the affected vein, resulting in fibrosis and obliteration of the lumen. Sclerotherapy has largely been overtaken in popularity by banding, where an 'O' ring is applied to the haemorrhoid in order to strangulate it. Care must be taken to ensure correct placement of the ring above the dentate line, which is insensate. Application beneath this line would be extremely painful and the bands cannot be removed. Surgical haemorrhoidectomy is reserved for third-degree haemorrhoids. Lord's procedure, described as manual dilatation of the anus by inserting four fingers for four minutes, has historically been used to manage haemorrhoids, fissures and proctitis fugax. Due to the high incidence of post-procedure incontinence, it should no longer be performed.

2. A – DeLorme procedure

Rectal prolapses can either be partial or complete. Partial rectal prolapses involve prolapse of the rectal mucosa only. Palpation of the prolapse between the thumb and forefinger will determine that there is no muscle within the prolapse. Complete rectal prolapses include prolapse of both the rectal mucosa and muscle. It occurs most often in elderly females. Complete rectal prolapses result in faecal incontinence, due to stretching of the sphincter, along with mucus discharge. Partial prolapses are managed by excision of the redundant prolapsed mucosa. Complete prolapses are managed by surgical lifting of the prolapse. An example of this is DeLorme procedure, where the redundant mucosa is excised followed by placation (folding) of the muscle using sutures.

Edmond DeLorme, French surgeon (1847–1929).

3. H – Seton insertion

This woman has probably developed anal fistulae as a complication of inflammatory bowel disease. A fistula is defined as an abnormal connection between two epithelial surfaces. The only exception to this is an arteriovenous fistula, which is a connection between two endothelial surfaces. Anal fistulae result when an anal abscess ruptures into the anal canal. Patients present with a constant discharge from the external opening of the fistula. Goodsall's rule can be applied to the examination of anal fistulae. It states that if a fistula lies in the anterior half of the anal area (while the patient is in the lithotomy position) then it opens directly into the anal canal. However, if a fistula lies in the posterior half then it tracks around the anus to open in the midline posteriorly. The best way to delineate the anatomy of a fistula is by MRI scanning.

The treatment of anal fistulae depends on whether or not they pass through the puborectalis muscle of the anal sphincter. Inter-sphincteric fistulae (which lie below the puborectalis) are managed by laying open the fistula tract. Higher trans-sphincteric fistulae (which pass though the puborectalis) should not be laid open, due to the significant risk of subsequent faecal incontinence. Instead, a non-absorbable suture (or seton) is passed into the fistula tract and tied. This gradually cuts through the muscle, allowing it to heal by scarring.

4. D – Incision and drainage

This man appears to have developed a perianal abscess. A perianal abscess is a collection of pus next to the anus that results from infection of a hair follicle, sebaceous gland or a perianal haematoma. They are more common in people with inflammatory bowel disease or diabetes. Abscesses need to be treated by incision and drainage to prevent spontaneous internal rupture and fistula formation. An elliptical excision is made over the point of maximal fluctuance to release the abscess. Loculations should be broken down using digital manipulation within the cavity. Following curretage and a wash out, the cavity can be packed loosely and left to heal by secondary intention.

5. B – Diltiazem cream

This woman has developed an anal fissure. The management of painful anal fissures is with creams that relax the anal tone. Examples are diltiazem and glycerine trinitrate creams.

THEME 13: UPPER LIMB NERVE LESIONS

1. B – Axillary nerve

This man presents with an anterior shoulder dislocation. The axillary nerve wraps around the surgical neck of the humerus and is damaged in 5–10% of anterior dislocations. It can also be affected with fractures of the humeral neck. The axillary nerve supplies the deltoid muscle and gives rise to the lateral cutaneous nerve of the arm (which supplies sensation to the upper, outer arm). Axillary nerve lesions result in anaesthesia of the upper, outer arm (the 'regimental badge patch' area) and paralysis of the deltoid muscle, resulting in limited arm abduction. Before attempting reduction of the shoulder, axillary nerve function should be tested and documented by testing sensation of the upper outer arm. The arm cannot be abducted, but, if it is passively lifted above 90°, the arm can be held in abduction due to the action of the supraspinatus.

2. H – Proximal ulnar nerve

Supracondylar fractures can result in ulnar nerve lesions at the elbow (a proximal ulnar nerve lesion). Because the ulnar nerve supplies the flexors to the forearm, lesions of this nerve result in unopposed action of the forearm extensors, with the slight development of a claw-hand in the fourth and fifth digits (hyperextension of the metacarpophalangeal joints with flexion of the interphalangeal joints). Proximal ulnar nerve lesions also result in a loss of sensation to the ulnar side of the hand. The clawing that occurs with proximal ulnar nerve lesions is not as marked as that that occurs with distal lesions. This is because the flexor digitorum profundus, which is supplied by the proximal ulnar nerve, is intact in distal lesions, resulting in more flexion of the interphalangeal joints and an exacerbated flexion deformity.

3. E – Long thoracic nerve

The long thoracic nerve of Bell supplies the serratus anterior, a muscle that helps stabilize the scapula. It is formed from the three anterior rami of the spinal nerves C5, C6 and C7. The nerve can be damaged during breast and axillary surgery, radiotherapy, and axillary trauma. Lesions of the long thoracic nerve result in winging of the scapula, where the scapula becomes prominent on pushing the arms against resistance.

4. F – Lower brachial plexus

Lower brachial plexus injuries, also known as Klumpke palsy, involve the C8 and T1 nerve roots. They are often caused by breech birth injuries (when the baby's arm remains above its head) and when a person grabs something to break a fall. Patients present with a claw-hand in all digits (from paralysis of the intrinsic muscles of the hand) and sensory loss along the ulnar border of the forearm and hand.

Augusta Marie Dejerine-Klumpke, French neurologist (1859–1927).

5. A – Accessory nerve

The spinal root of the accessory nerve (cranial nerve XI) supplies the trapezius and sternocleidomastoid muscles. It can be damaged during dissections of the neck because of its superficial course. Features of accessory nerve palsy include weakness of shoulder shrugging and the inability to turn the head against a force applied by the examiner.

THEME 14: ANATOMY OF HERNIAS

1. G – Pantaloon

A pantaloon hernia is a type of direct inguinal hernia where the hernial sac straddles the inferior epigastric vessels.

2. B – Gluteal

A gluteal hernia is one that protrudes through the greater sciatic foramen, a foramen in the pelvis that is bounded by the greater sciatic notch, the sacrospinous ligament and the sacrotuberous ligament. A sciatic hernia is one that passes through the lesser sciatic foramen.

3. E – Maydl

A Maydl hernia is one that contains a 'W'-loop of intestine within the hernial sac and where the middle segment of the loop becomes strangulated.

Karel Maydl, Austrian surgeon (1853–1903).

4. D – Lumbar

There are two types of lumbar hernia. A Petit hernia passes through the inferior lumbar triangle of the posterolateral wall, which is bounded by the external oblique muscle, the latissimus dorsi and the iliac crest below. A Grynfeltt hernia passes through the superior lumbar triangle, which is bounded by the 12th rib above, the sacrospinalis muscle medially and the internal oblique muscle laterally.

Jean Louis Petit, French surgeon (1674–1750).

Joseph Grynfeltt, French surgeon (1840–1913).

5. A – Amyand

An Amyand (or Garengoff) hernia is one that contains the appendix within the hernial sac.

Obturator hernias pass through the obturator canal in the upper thigh and usually occur in elderly women. These hernias typically incarcerate and interfere with the obturator nerve, which supplies sensation to the medial thigh. The Howship–Romberg sign, where pain is elicited along the medial aspect of the thigh on abduction, extension or internal rotation of the knee, is positive in 50% of cases. A Littré hernia describes the hernial protrusion of a Meckel intestinal diverticulum.

Claudius Amyand, English surgeon (1680–1740).

John Howship, English surgeon (1781–1841).

Moritz Heinrich Romberg, German neurologist (1795–1873).

Alexis Littré, French anatomist (1654–1726).

THEME 15: MANAGEMENT OF COMMON FRACTURES

1. F – Manipulation anaesthesia

This woman has a Colles fracture that needs to be manipulated under anaesthesia before being immobilized in a forearm and wrist plaster. Although not part of the options available here, an adequate position may be achieved by reducing the fracture in the emergency department under light sedation. Key aspects to note include whether the fracture is on the dominant side, the level of function required (e.g. the patient is a concert pianist!) and whether the fracture is intra- or extra-articular.

2. B – Broad arm sling

Fractured clavicles are common in children and young adults. Clavicles most often break at the junction of the middle and outer thirds. If displacement occurs, the lateral fragment is displaced downward and medially by the weight of the arm and the medial fragment is held up by the sternomastoid muscle. Management is by using a broad arm sling for 2 weeks, with active exercises after 1 week. Union is good, but in adults a slight deformity (thickening) is usual. Operative fixation may occasionally be indicated in comminuted fractures or those which are widely displaced (showing signs of skin tenting).

3. C – Dynamic hip screw

Intertrochanteric fractures of the femur are extracapsular and do not compromise the blood supply to the femoral head. The ideal method of fixation of these fractures is a dynamic hip screw, as it allows good fixation and early mobilization. The dynamic hip screw consists of a plate, which is fixed to the lateral aspect of the femur, and a screw that passes through the plate at an oblique angle passing parallel to the femoral neck and into the centre of the femoral head. As the patient's weight passes through the prosthesis, the fracture site will remodel as the femoral head is compacted down along a single plane.

4. H – Plaster cast

Fractures of the humeral shaft require neither perfect reduction nor immobilization, and contact over a third of the area is sufficient. Management is by forming a plaster cast to maintain alignment. If there is significant displacement then manipulation under anaesthesia is required first. Exercises should be carried out as soon as possible.

5. A – Analgesia alone

This woman has developed a march fracture in the second metatarsal. Management is symptomatic, as these fractures heal spontaneously.

THEME 16: DIAGNOSIS OF VASCULAR DISEASE

1. K – Takayasu arteritis

Takayasu arteritis (also known as pulseless disease) is a rare vasculitis characterized by granulomatous inflammation of the aorta and its major branches. Features include hypertension, arm claudication, absent pulses, bruits and visual disturbance (transient ambylopia and blindness). Patients also present with systemic illness (malaise, fever, night sweats and weight loss). It is most common in younger Asian women. Diagnosis is by angiography, which shows narrowing of the aorta and its major branches. Management is with steroids, but the condition is progressive and death occurs within a few years.

Mikito Takayasu, Japanese ophthalmologist (1860–1938).

2. B – Deep vein thrombosis (DVT)

Venous thromboembolism occurs in response to three factors as described by Virchow's triad: (1) endothelial damage (e.g. smoking or previous DVT), (2) reduced venous flow (e.g. immobility or obstruction to flow) and (3) hypercoagulability. DVT is a relatively common complication in surgical patients, occurring in 50% of patients undergoing major abdominal surgery if no prophylactic measures are taken. Consequently the risk of developing thrombo-embolic disease should be assessed for each patient and weighed up against the risk of bleeding. The vast majority of surgical patients will receive a mixture of physical thromboprophylaxis (TED stockings and intermittent pneumatic compression boots) and chemical prophylaxis (low-molecular-weight heparin). Risk factors include increasing age, previous thromboembolism, immobility, obesity, pregnancy, contraceptive pill use and thrombophilic states (e.g. factor V Leiden mutation, proteins C or S deficiency, and antithrombin III deficiency). For those patients at high risk of bleeding, low-molecular-weight heparin may be inappropriate because of its comparatively long half-life. IV heparin is a useful alternative as its half-life is much shorter and can be reversed if necessary with protamine.

DVT may be asymptomatic, but patients often present with pain erythema and swelling in the calf, along with mild pyrexia. Homans sign, described as increased pain on dorsiflexion of the foot, may be present, but is a non-specific sign. Phlegmasia caerulia dolens is a painful, purple, oedematous leg secondary to ileofemoral DVT. DVT can embolize to result in pulmonary embolism.

Rudolf Ludwig Karl Virchow, German pathologist (1821–1902).

John Homans, American surgeon (1877–1954).

3. E – Klippel–Trénaunay syndrome

Klippel–Trénaunay syndrome is a congenital vascular malformation that presents with multiple port-wine stains, varicose veins on the lateral aspect of the thigh and hypertrophy of the bones and soft tissues of one leg. Patients are predisposed to multiple deep vein thromboses. Sturge-Weber syndrome is a congenital disorder characterized by port-wine stains in the trigeminal distribution with epilepsy.

Maurice Klippel, French neurologist (1858–1942).

Paul Trénaunay, French neurologist (b1875).

4. F – Raynaud disease

Raynaud disease is an idiopathic condition with episodic digital vasospasm precipitated by a cold environment. As a result, the affected fingers or toes become white and may be painful. If vasospasm persists, the fingers become blue (from cyanosis) and subsequently turn red (reactive hyperaemia). If features of Raynaud disease occur secondary to another medical condition then it is known as Raynaud syndrome. Such conditions include scleroderma, lupus, Buerger disease, vibration injury and frostbite.

Maurice Raynaud, French physician (1834–1881).

5. D – Intermittent claudication

Intermittent claudication is a cramping pain that occurs with exercise and is relieved by rest. (Pain that is present on standing and is relieved by bending over or sitting is indicative of spinal stenosis.) Intermittent claudication occurs secondary to atherosclerotic stenosis or occlusion of the arteries proximal to the affected muscle. For example, calf claudication is secondary to superficial femoral artery lesions, and buttock claudication occurs with internal or common iliac artery stenosis. Bilateral buttock claudication associated with impotence is known as Leriche syndrome and is due to bilateral internal iliac disease.

Claudication, from Latin *claudere* = to limp; this word derives from the name of the Roman Emperor Claudius, who is said to have walked with a limp.

René Leriche, French surgeon (1879–1955).

Practice Paper 4: Questions

THEME 1: DIAGNOSIS OF DYSPHAGIA

Options

A. Bulbar palsy
B. Chagas disease
C. Diffuse oesophageal spasm
D. External oesophageal compression
E. Gastro-oesophageal reflux disease
F. Myasthenia gravis
G. Oesophageal candidiasis
H. Oesophageal carcinoma
I. Oesophageal web
J. Pseudobulbar palsy
K. Scleroderma

For each of the following people presenting with dysphagia, select the most likely diagnosis. Each option may be used once, more than once or not at all.

1. A 46-year-old woman presents with intermittent severe retrosternal chest pains that occur soon after eating and are accompanied by dysphagia. She complains of no other symptoms. An ECG shows no acute abnormality and cardiac enzymes are normal.
2. A 72-year-old man presents with a 3-month history of dysphagia and odynophagia. This initially occurred with solids, but he is now finding it difficult to drink liquids. Over the past months, he has lost 12 kg in weight. Examination is unremarkable.
3. A 44-year-old man, who has recently arrived in the country from Brazil, presents with a 5-month history of dysphagia for solids and liquids. He is otherwise fit and well, and examination demonstrates no other abnormality. A chest X-ray shows an air–fluid level behind the heart.
4. A 36-year-old man presents with a 4-month history of increasing difficulty in swallowing. You notice that his speech is a little slurred, and his wife tells you that this is a new development. On examination, his tongue is wasted and shows fasciculations.
5. A 42-year-old man presents with retrosterwnal pain and dysphagia. He is currently on a course of prednisolone for an exacerbation of

inflammatory bowel disease. On examination, you notice multiple white lesions in his mouth that rub off easily.

THEME 2: SHOCK

Options

A. Anaphylactic shock
B. Cardiogenic shock
C. Class I hypovolaemic shock
D. Class II hypovolaemic shock
E. Class III hypovolaemic shock
F. Class IV hypovolaemic shock
G. Neurogenic shock
H. Septic shock
I. Spinal shock

For each of the following scenarios, select the most likely type of shock. Each option may be used once, more than once or not at all.

1. A 27-year-old man presents following a drinking binge with four episodes of haematemesis. On examination, he is drowsy and confused. His pulse is 96/min, blood pressure 130/70 mmHg and urine output 60 mL in the first hour.
2. A 54-year-old man presents with erythema and pain in his right calf. On examination, the area is diffuse, warm and around 5 cm in size. His heart rate is 120/min, blood pressure 100/65 mmHg and respiratory rate 30/min. His temperature is 38.5°C.
3. A 67-year-old diabetic presents with a 3-hour history of feeling very unwell. On examination, he is cool and clammy, and his jugular venous pulse is elevated. His pulse is 110/min and blood pressure 90/50 mmHg.
4. A 24-year-old man presents following a road traffic accident with bilateral femoral fractures. On examination, he appears pale. His pulse is 130/min, blood pressure 80/58 mmHg and respiratory rate 30/min. His urine output was measured as 30 mL over 3 hours.
5. A 42-year-old woman is brought to hospital following a road traffic accident. On arrival in hospital, she suddenly becomes faint. On examination, her peripheries feel warm and dry. Her pulse is 40/min and blood pressure 82/48 mmHg.

THEME 3: MANAGEMENT OF CHEST TRAUMA

Options

A. Analgesia and respiratory support
B. Apply a three-sided occlusive dressing
C. Arteriography
D. Cardiopulmonary resuscitation
E. Chest drain insertion
F. Chest X-ray

G. Immediate thoracotomy
H. Needle aspiration
I. Needle thoracocentesis
J. Pericardiocentesis

For each of the following people presenting after trauma, select the most appropriate management. Each option may be used once, more than once or not at all.

1. A 27-year-old man is involved in a motorcycle accident. He develops shortness of breath, with a respiratory rate of 32/min and a heart rate of 110/min. On examination, you notice some paradoxical movements of the chest wall.
2. A 35-year-old woman is brought to the emergency department following a car crash. On arrival, her blood pressure is 110/50 mmHg, heart rate 92/min and respiratory rate 28/min. On examination, there is decreased air entry on the right side, as well as dullness to percussion.
3. A 42-year-old man is stabbed in the left side of his chest during a bar brawl. On arrival at the emergency department, his blood pressure is 80/42 mmHg and his heart rate 112/min. The jugular veins are visibly engorged and the heart sounds are barely audible on auscultation.
4. A 21-year-old woman is involved in a road traffic accident. When the paramedics arrive, she has a heart rate of 122/min, a respiratory rate of 32/min and a blood pressure of 86/42 mmHg. On examination, there are absent breath sounds and hyper-resonance to percussion on the left side. The trachea is deviated to the right.
5. A 32-year-old man is stabbed in the right side of his chest. He struggles to the hospital. On arrival, he is in some respiratory distress. On examination, there is decreased air entry and hyper-resonance to percussion on the right side. The trachea is not deviated. The doctor notes the presence of a sucking wound in the right chest.

THEME 4: DIAGNOSIS OF ABDOMINAL PAIN

Options

A. Acute appendicitis
B. Acute pancreatitis
C. Chronic pancreatitis
D. Diverticulitis
E. Ectopic pregnancy
F. Irritable bowel syndrome
G. Mesenteric angina
H. Pelvic abscess
I. Pelvic inflammatory disease
J. Perforated peptic ulcer
K. Subphrenic abscess

For each of the following people presenting with abdominal pain, select the most likely diagnosis. Each option may be used once, more than once or not at all.

1. A 23-year-old woman presents with a 3-day history of left iliac fossa pain and nausea. Further questioning reveals that she is also suffering pain on micturation. On examination, there is tenderness and guarding in the left iliac fossa as well as some tenderness in the right upper quadrant. Her temperature is 37.6°C.
2. A 68-year-old woman with a history of osteoarthritis presents with acute severe abdominal pain and vomiting. On examination, the abdomen is rigid and bowel sounds are absent.
3. A 42-year-old woman presents with an 8-month history of abdominal discomfort that is improved following defaecation. She complains of a regular change in her bowel habit, alternating between constipation and loose motions. On examination, her abdomen is soft and nontender. There are no obvious masses, and bowel sounds are present.
4. A 44-year-old man presents with recurrent episodes of severe epigastric pain that radiates to his back and is improved on leaning forwards. On examination, he is jaundiced, with guarding in his epigastrium, but there is no evidence of haemorrhage. Observations are stable. Routine bloods are sent off, and the amylase returns at 248 IU/L.
5. A 68-year-old woman undergoes a laparotomy for a perforated diverticulum. A few days later, she develops pain in the left upper quadrant that radiates to the shoulder, nausea, vomiting and rigors. Her temperature is 38.9°C.

THEME 5: HAND DISORDERS

Options

A. de Quervain tenovaginitis
B. Dupuytren contracture
C. Gamekeeper's thumb
D. Ganglion
E. Mallet finger
F. Mid-palmar space infection
G. Paronychia
H. Tendon sheath infection
I. Thenar space infection
J. Trigger finger
K. Whitlow

For each of the following people presenting with hand problems, select the most likely diagnosis. Each option may be used once, more than once or not at all.

1. An 18-year-old man presents with a painless swelling on the dorsum of the left hand. There is a smooth, tense swelling around 2 cm in diameter that is not attached to the overlying skin.
2. A 42-year-old woman presents with pain in her right wrist. On examination, there is tenderness localized to the dorsoradial aspect of the wrist that is exacerbated by thumb movement.
3. A 54-year-old man presents with problems with his right index finger. He reports that it often gets stuck when he bends his finger, and he has to manually straighten it. He denies any history of trauma to the area.
4. A 62-year-old man presents with a long history of fixed flexion deformity in his hand. On closer inspection, there is flexion of the right fourth digit. On palpation, the palmar aponeurosis can be felt to be thickened.
5. A 26-year-old man attends the emergency department with pain in his left palm. On examination, the lateral half of the palm is swollen, erythematous and very tender. The patient admits to unintentionally cutting himself on the hand last week.

THEME 6: DIAGNOSIS OF BILIARY TRACT DISEASE

Options

A. Acute cholecystitis
B. Ascending cholangitis
C. Biliary colic
D. Cholangiocarcinoma
E. Choledocholithiasis
F. Chronic cholecystitis
G. Empyema of the gallbladder
H. Gallbladder perforation
I. Gallstone ileus
J. Mirizzi syndrome
K. Primary sclerosing cholangitis

For each of the following scenarios, select the most likely diagnosis. Each option may be used once, more than once or not at all.

1. An 82-year-old woman presents with worsening jaundice and weight loss. An abdominal ultrasound shows dilatation of the common bile duct, and a subsequent magnetic resonance cholangiopancreatogram (MRCP) confirms an irregular stenosing lesion in the common bile duct.
2. A 48-year-old woman presents with a 3-day history of abdominal pain. On examination, she is clinically jaundiced and tender in the right upper quadrant, but no masses are palpable. An ultrasound scan confirms the presence of biliary stones and intrahepatic duct dilatation. An MRCP shows a gallstone within the gallbladder pressing on the common bile duct.
3. A 58-year-old woman with known gallstones presents with a 12-month history of indigestion attacks and flatulence. Symptoms occur after meals

and can last up to an hour. On examination, she is obese but shows no signs of jaundice or anaemia. Her abdomen is soft and non-tender.

4. A 32-year-old man with ulcerative colitis presents with a 4-week history of worsening jaundice. He denies any pain, fevers or nausea. On examination, his abdomen is soft. An abdominal ultrasound shows dilatation of the intrahepatic biliary tree but a normal common bile duct.
5. A 38-year-old woman presents with a 48-hour history of right upper quadrant pain, nausea and vomiting. On examination, she is clinically jaundiced and her temperature is 38.5°C. An abdominal ultrasound shows multiple stones in the gallbladder and a common bile duct diameter of 9 mm.

THEME 7: INVESTIGATION OF UROLOGICAL DISEASE

Options

A. Anterograde urethrogram
B. Bladder scan and urethral catheterisation
C. CT scan
D. Cystoscopy and retrograde ureteric stent
E. Intravenous urogram
F. Percutaneous nephrostomy
G. Three-way catheter and irrigation
H. Transrectal ultrasound and biopsy
I. Ultrasound scan of abdomen
J. Urgent surgical exploration

For each of the following scenarios, select the next most appropriate investigation. Each option may be used once, more than once or not at all.

1. A 22-year-old man presents to the emergency department after being hit by a reversing car. He has an episode of macroscopic haematuria, but abdominal and per rectum examinations show no other abnormality. His blood pressure is 114/74 mmHg and his pulse 86/min.
2. A 74-year-old man presents with acute-onset suprapubic pain and an inability to pass urine. On examination, he is visibly uncomfortable and the bladder is percussable 6 cm above the pubis.
3. A 37-year-old man was cycling home when his bike skidded on ice and he crashed into a post box. On admission to the emergency department, he has complained of an inability to pass urine and on examination there is blood at the external urethral meatus.
4. A 61-year-old man presents with sudden-onset left loin pain that radiates to his groin. He has been unable to pass urine over the last 24 hours. He has a history of a right nephrectomy for a renal cell carcinoma. A spiral CT scan confirms the presence of a 6 mm stone at the left vesicoureteric junction and a left hydronephrosis.

5. A 58-year-old man is referred to the clinic by his general practitioner with a prostate-specific antigen level of 14.0 ng/mL. He has no other symptoms. Abdominal examination shows no abnormality, but an enlarged, hard, irregular prostate gland is palpable per rectum.

THEME 8: LOWER GASTROINTESTINAL HAEMORRHAGE

Options

A. Anal fissure
B. Angiodysplasia
C. Colorectal cancer
D. Crohn's disease
E. Diverticular disease
F. Diverticulitis
G. Haemorrhoids
H. Infective colitis
I. Ischaemic colitis
J. Ulcerative colitis

For each of the following people presenting with bleeding, select the most appropriate investigation. Each option may be used once, more than once or not at all.

1. An 86-year-old woman presents with bright-red rectal bleeding. She had two previous similar episodes in the last month. The patient denies abdominal pain or any other symptoms. A barium enema and colonoscopy are performed, but no abnormality is detected.
2. A 38-year-old woman presents with a 2-day history of increased frequency of motions. She describes these motions as loose and blood-stained. The patient also complains of generalized abdominal tenderness and vomiting. On examination of the abdomen, there is no guarding or masses. A digital rectal examination is unremarkable.
3. A 62-year-old woman presents with a single episode of fresh rectal bleeding. She denies having any abdominal pain, fever, weight loss or history of rectal bleeding. On further questioning, you ascertain a 6-month history of worsening constipation and left iliac fossa pain that is relieved by defecation.
4. A 68-year-old man attends his general practice with a 3-week history of alternating constipation and diarrhoea. He used to open his bowels once daily. On further questioning, he admits to passing fresh blood occasionally per rectum. A digital rectal exam reveals haemorrhoids but nothing else.
5. A 17-year-old girl presents with a 4-week history of right iliac fossa pain that has become worse over the last couple of days. She admits to the occasional passage of blood and mucus over this period. On examination, a mass can be palpated in the right iliac fossa.

THEME 9: TUMOUR MARKERS

Options

A. α-fetoprotein
B. β-hCG
C. CA 125
D. CA 15-3
E. CA 19-9
F. Calcitonin
G. Carcinoembryonic antigen
H. Paraproteins
I. Prostate-specific antigen
J. S-100

For each of the following presentations, select the most appropriate tumour marker. Each option may be used once, more than once or not at all.

1. A 47-year-old woman presents with a 3 cm firm lump in the left breast that is fixed to the overlying skin.
2. A 76-year-old man complains of new constipation. He has a history of passing fresh blood mixed with his stools and has recently lost weight.
3. A 68-year-old man presents with difficulty passing urine and dribbling at the end of the stream.
4. A 34-year-old woman presents with a 1 cm flat, brown lesion on her left leg. On examination, the lesion is irregularly pigmented and occasionally itches and bleeds.
5. A 62-year-old woman presents with jaundice that has been worsening over the previous weeks. She denies having any pain. On examination, the gallbladder is palpable.

THEME 10: INVESTIGATION OF BREAST DISEASE

Options

A. Aspirate culture
B. Aspirate cytology
C. Core biopsy
D. CT scan
E. Fine-needle aspiration cytology
F. Magnetic resonance imaging
G. Mammography
H. No further investigation
I. Ultrasound scan

For each of the following people presenting with breast disease, select the next step in the investigation. Each option may be used once, more than once or not at all.

1. A 34-year-old woman presents to the breast clinic with a history of lumpiness and tenderness in both breasts that is worse in the days prior to menstruation. An ultrasound scan reveals multiple small cysts bilaterally, and a tissue sample shows fibrosis and epithelial hyperplasia.
2. A 28-year-old woman presents with a 1 cm soft lump in her right breast that appeared suddenly last week. The lesion is painless and there is no other abnormality on examination.
3. A 42-year-old woman presents to the breast clinic with a hard 2 cm lump in the upper outer quadrant of the left breast associated with axillary lymphadenopathy. She has a history of bilateral breast augmentation for cosmetic reasons. A mammogram is performed, but the resulting image is hazy and the radiologist cannot confidently delineate any lesions.
4. A 52-year-old woman attends the breast clinic with a 4 cm lump in her left breast. A fine-needle aspiration was performed and the cells sent for cytology. The resulting report notes the presence of dysplastic cells.
5. A 45-year-old woman complains of a lump in her right breast that has been present for some time. An ultrasound scan reveals a breast cyst, and this is aspirated under ultrasound guidance. The aspirate is found to be blood-stained.

THEME 11: PENILE CONDITIONS

Options

A. Circinate balanitis
B. Erectile dysfunction
C. Keratoderma blennorrhagicum
D. Paraphimosis
E. Penile cancer
F. Peyronie disease
G. Phimosis
H. Priapism

For each of the following men presenting with genital abnormalities, select the most appropriate diagnosis. Each option may be used once, more than once or not at all.

1. A 36-year-old man presents with a weak stream on micturation. He complains of no other symptoms. On examination, the foreskin is tight, thickened and closely adherent to the glans. It is pale in colour.
2. A 28-year-old man presents to the general practitioner with pain on passing water and pain in his knee. On examination, you notice his eyes are red. There are raised, erythematous lesions on the glans of the penis.
3. A 60-year-old man presents with a history of pain on erection. He also describes difficulty with sexual intercourse. On examination, you notice an abnormal ventral curvature of the penis.
4. A 37-year-old man presents to the emergency department with a painful erection that he has had for 6 hours and cannot get rid of.

5. An 80-year-old man presents with a painful ulcer on his glans. On examination, there is a bloody purulent discharge from the ulcer and inguinal lymphadenopathy is palpable bilaterally.

THEME 12: CUTANEOUS MALIGNANCIES

Options

A. Acral lentiginous melanoma
B. Actinic keratosis
C. Amelanotic melanoma
D. Basal cell carcinoma
E. Bowen disease
F. Keratoacanthoma
G. Lentigo maligna melanoma
H. Nodular melanoma
I. Squamous cell carcinoma
J. Superficial spreading malignant melanoma

For each of the following people presenting with skin lesions, select the most likely diagnosis. Each option may be used once, more than once or not at all.

1. A 32-year-old woman presents with a flat, irregular pigmented lesion on her leg. This has grown in size in the past month and occasionally bleeds.
2. A 67-year-old man presents with a lesion on his arm that first appeared last month but has grown rapidly since. On examination, there is a 2 cm nodule with a central necrotic plug.
3. A 64-year-old woman presents with a large pinky-brown lesion on her lower leg. On examination, the lesion is 4 cm, flat and scaly, with an irregular border.
4. A 77-year-old man presents with a lesion on his upper ear that has been present for months but has begun to ulcerate. On examination, there is a non-pigmented hyperkeratotic, crusty lesion with raised everted edges on the pinna.
5. An 80-year-old woman has a large pigmented lesion on her left cheek that she has had for some years. She presents to her general practitioner because a thickened, pigmented, irregular lesion is growing on the edge of the previous one.

THEME 13: MANAGEMENT OF ENDOCRINE DISEASE

Options

A. Iodine-131
B. Carbimazole
C. Desmopressin
D. Hydrocortisone and fludrocortisone
E. Octreotide

F. Spironolactone
G. Surgical resection and radiotherapy
H. Thyroxine alone
I. Total thyroidectomy and thyroxine

For each of the following presentations of endocrine disease, select the best management option. Each option may be used once, more than once or not at all.

1. A 72-year-old woman presents with worsening difficulty in swallowing food. Because of this, she is finding it hard to eat. On examination, you note a large, hard, irregular mass in the neck that is attached to the overlying skin. She tells you that the lump has been present for a month and has been growing rapidly.
2. A 32-year-old woman presents to her general practitioner with a 1-month history of worsening diarrhoea and heat intolerance. On examination, she has a mild tremor and bulging eyes. She would like treatment for her condition, but warns you that she is pregnant.
3. A 26-year-old man attends his first outpatient clinic following a head injury that resulted in hospitalization last month. He complains of recent polyuria and polydipsia but no other symptoms. His blood pressure is 120/85 mmHg and his heart rate 72/min.
4. An 18-year-old woman attends her general practitioner with a lump in her neck that has been present for a few weeks. On examination, the lump is smooth and non-tender and moves up with swallowing but not on tongue protrusion. Cervical lymphadenopathy is also noted.
5. A 14-year-old girl attends paediatric outpatients following meningococcal septicaemia a few weeks previously. She complains of feeling tired, weak and having a poor appetite. She feels dizzy when standing up from a sitting position. Her blood tests show sodium 127 mmol/L and potassium 5.4 mmol/L.

THEME 14: EYE DISEASE

Options

A. Acute closed-angle glaucoma
B. Anterior uveitis
C. Blepharitis
D. Conjunctivitis
E. Ectropion
F. Entropion
G. Episcleritis
H. Hyphaema
I. Scleritis
J. Scleromalacia
K. Stye

For each of the following presentations of eye disease, select the most likely diagnosis. Each option may be used once, more than once or not at all.

1. A 32-year-old man presents to the general practitioner with bilateral painful red eyes. He has had three such episodes over the last month. He also complains of stiffness in his lower back. On examination, there is conjunctival injection around the iris, and the pupils have an irregular outline.
2. A 46-year-old woman presents with painless reddening of her eyes. She is also complaining of pain in the small joints of her hands that has been worsening over the previous year.
3. A 66-year-old woman presents with sudden onset, severe pain in her right eye. She admits to poor vision, nausea and vomiting. On examination, the eye is inflamed and very tender and firm to palpation. The pupil of the affected eye is fixed and ovoid in shape.
4. A 35-year-old woman presents with bilateral itchy eyes. On examination, you notice that her eyelids and eyes are red and itchy. There is some crusting on the lid margins and both eyelids are depleted of eyelashes.
5. A 42-year-old woman presents to the general practitioner with discomfort and reddening of her left eye. It has been present for 2 days and is associated with a purulent discharge.

THEME 15: PREOPERATIVE MORBIDITY

Options

A. ASA grade I
B. ASA grade IE
C. ASA grade II
D. ASA grade IIE
E. ASA grade III
F. ASA grade IIIE
G. ASA grade IV
H. ASA grade IVE
I. ASA grade V
J. ASA grade VE

For each of the following scenarios, select the most appropriate ASA grade. Each option may be used once, more than once or not at all.

1. A 38-year-old man with medication-controlled inflammatory bowel disease who is about to have an inguinal hernia repair.
2. A 43-year-old man with tablet-controlled hypertension who is about to have his varicose veins ligated.
3. A 38-year-old woman with severe asthma who regularly needs acute admission and who is to have an elective cholecystectomy.

4. A 67-year-old woman has regular dialysis for chronic renal failure. She wants to have bilateral knee replacements for osteoarthritis.
5. A 76-year-old man who presents with features suggesting a ruptured abdominal aortic aneurysm is taken to theatre for an emergency repair.

THEME 16: BONE TUMOURS

Options

A. Chondrosarcoma
B. Enchondroma
C. Ewing sarcoma
D. Osteochondroma
E. Osteoclastoma (giant cell tumour)
F. Osteoid osteoma
G. Osteolytic bony metastases
H. Osteoporotic bony metastases
I. Osteosarcoma

For each of the following presentations, select the most likely diagnosis. Each option may be used once, more than once or not at all.

1. A 47-year-old man presents with an asymmetric swelling on the right lower rib cage. On examination, the swelling is tender. A chest X-ray demonstrates localized bone destruction at the lower costal margin, with areas of calcification.
2. A 15-year-old boy attends the emergency department with pain in the lower left leg and fever. On examination, there is a tender, irregular swelling at the tibia. X-ray of the leg shows a lytic lesion with a laminated periosteal reaction.
3. A 22-year-old man presents with an enlarging, painful lesion in his distal femur. An X-ray of the femur shows an ill-defined lesion with calcification associated with elevation of the periosteum.
4. A 20-year-old man presents with a 2-week history of pain in his thigh that is worse at night. The pain is relieved promptly by non-steroidal anti-inflammatories. An X-ray of the affected thigh demonstrates a radiolucent area within the femur, surrounded by a ring of dense bone.
5. A 72-year-old man develops a painful, enlarging mass in his left tibia. An X-ray of the leg shows periosteal elevation and anterior bowing of the tibia. A chest X-ray reveals multiple, discrete lesions in both lung fields.

THEME 17: MANAGEMENT OF ARTERIAL DISEASE

Options

A. Amputation
B. Aorto-bifemoral bypass graft
C. Best medical therapy
D. Embolectomy

E. Endarterectomy left side
F. Endarterectomy right side
G. Fasciotomy
H. Femoro-popliteal bypass
I. Percutaneous balloon angioplasty
J. Thrombolysis

For each of the following scenarios, select the most appropriate management plan. Each option may be used once, more than once or not at all.

1. A 55-year-old man presents with right-sided cramping pain in his calf on exertion. The pain lasts 2 minutes and is relieved by rest. On examination, there is no abnormality in the lower limbs and all pulses are palpable.
2. A 62-year-old man presents with sudden-onset pain in the left lower leg. The patient has a past medical history of atrial fibrillation and was recently admitted with a stroke. On examination, the left leg is cold and painful and the pedal pulses are not palpable.
3. A 53-year-old man was admitted to the emergency department with an acutely ischaemic limb that was managed by surgical embolectomy. A few hours after the operation, the patient complains of worsening pain in his leg. On examination, the affected leg is slightly swollen and the patient experiences severe pain on dorsiflexion of the foot.
4. A 62-year-old man with diabetes and a long history of peripheral vascular disease is in hospital for management of an infected lower limb arterial ulcer. One morning on the ward round, you notice that the big toe on his left foot is black.
5. A 72-year-old woman presents with sudden-onset right-sided facial weakness lasting 12 hours followed by complete resolution. She denies any visual disturbance. Carotid Doppler ultrasound scans show bilateral carotid artery stenosis of 85%.

Practice Paper 4: Answers

THEME 1: DIAGNOSIS OF DYSPHAGIA

1. C – Diffuse oesophageal spasm

Diffuse oesophageal spasm, also known as 'nutcracker oesophagus', is an idiopathic condition characterized by intermittent spasm of the distal half of the oesophagus without any structural stenosis. Patients present with severe retrosternal chest pain lasting 30 minutes with or without dysphagia. Symptom frequency can vary from every few days to every time the patient eats. A barium swallow in active disease will show diffuse spasm, known as the 'corkscrew oesophagus'; however, as symptoms are intermittent, barium studies are often normal. Manometry will show prolonged, powerful oesophageal contractions induced by swallowing.

2. H – Oesophageal carcinoma

A history of rapidly progressive dysphagia with weight loss in a patient of this age (60–80 years) suggests a diagnosis of oesophageal carcinoma. Oesophageal carcinomas are mostly of the squamous cell type (worldwide), and risk factors for development include male sex, smoking, achalasia, alcohol use, coeliac disease and Chinese origin. Squamous cell carcinomas of the oesophagus occur most frequently in the mid-oesophagus, and spread of tumours is to local structures, such as the trachea and recurrent laryngeal nerve (blood metastases occur late). In the UK, adenocarcinoma is the more commonly seen. The diagnosis of oesophageal carcinoma is by endoscopy and biopsy, with a CT scan performed later to stage the disease. A barium swallow will show an irregular filling defect. Treatment is by oesophagectomy with re-anastomosis of the stomach to the upper oesophagus. A number of different approaches have been described, the principal ones being the Ivor Lewis, McKeown, and transhiatal. Oesophagectomy can now be performed laparoscopically in specialist centres. Unresectable tumours may be given palliative stenting or radiotherapy to improve dysphagia. Oesophageal tumours have a poor prognosis. Oesophageal adenocarcinoma can occur in a background of Barrett oesophagus.

3. B – Chagas disease

This man from South America presents with features similar to achalasia, but, given his country of origin, the diagnosis is likely to be Chagas disease. Chagas disease is a tropical parasitic disease of South America that is caused by the protozoan *Trypanosoma cruzi,* which is transmitted to humans by so-called 'assassin bugs'. In the acute stage of the disease, a skin nodule occurs at the site of inoculation (chagoma), along with fever, anorexia and lymphadenopathy. After a long asymptomatic period, patients can develop symptoms such as dysphagia (from destruction of the oesophageal myenteric plexus and a subsequent halt of peristalsis) and cardiomyopathy. It is thought that Charles Darwin contracted and eventually died from Chagas disease.

Carlos Chagas, Brazilian physician (1879–1934).

4. A – Bulbar palsy

Bulbar palsy is a lower motor neurone lesion of the cranial nerves of the medulla (9, 10, 11 and 12). Lower motor neurone lesions are characterized by hypotonicity and hyporeflexia, and features of a bulbar palsy include dysphagia, dysarthria, a weak fasciculating tongue and a diminished jaw jerk. Causes of a bulbar palsy include motor neurone disease, Guillain-Barré syndrome and myasthenia gravis. A pseudobulbar palsy is an upper motor neurone lesion (i.e. hypertonicity and hyperreflexia) characterized by dysphagia and dysarthria along with a small, spastic tongue and a brisk jaw jerk. Causes of a pseudobulbar palsy include motor neurone disease, multiple sclerosis, brainstem tumour and brainstem stroke.

5. G – Oesophageal candidiasis

This man with white oral lesions, dysphagia and recent steroid use has probably developed oesophageal candidiasis. Infection of the oesophagus by *Candida albicans* occurs most often in patients who are either immunosuppressed (e.g. AIDS or steroid use) or have recently used antibiotics. Patients often complain of dysphagia, odynophagia and a hoarse voice. Oesophageal candidiasis can be treated with antifungals such as fluconazole, nystatin or amphotericin.

THEME 2: SHOCK

There are five main types of shock: hypovolaemic, neurogenic, cardiogenic, septic and anaphylactic. Hypovolaemic shock can further be divided into classes I–IV as follows:

Class I	(15% loss) respiratory rate (RR) < 20 breaths/min, heart rate (HR) < 100 beats/min, blood pressure (BP) normal, urine output (UO) >30 mL/h
Class II	(15–30% loss) RR 20–30, HR 100–120, BP normal, UO 20–30
Class III	(30–40% loss) RR 30–40, HR 120–140, BP decreased, UO 5–20
Class IV	(>40% loss) RR > 40, HR > 140, BP decreased, UO < 5

The classes of the different stages of shock can be remembered easily as they follow the same scoring system of tennis; namely:

Class I	0–15%	Love–15
Class II	15–30%	15–30
Class III	30–40%	30–40
Class IV	>40%	Game

1. C – Class I hypovolaemic shock

This patient presents with haematemesis that is probably secondary to a Mallory-Weiss tear. His drowsiness is likely to be secondary to alcohol consumption rather than blood loss (although the absence of a significant head injury cannot be assumed). The normal heart rate, blood pressure and urine output suggest a class I hypovolaemia.

2. H – Septic shock

This patient appears to have cellulitis with resulting septic shock. Features of septic shock include warm skin, pyrexia, tachycardia, bounding pulse and hypotension. An arterial blood gas may determine a lactic acidosis. The features of septic shock are induced by the inflammatory response, although there may not necessarily be an infective focus (e.g. pancreatitis).

3. B – Cardiogenic shock

This diabetic patient has presented with a silent myocardial infarction with resulting cardiogenic shock. Cardiogenic shock is defined as hypotension with tissue hypoperfusion despite adequate ventricular filling. It is due to a failure of the ventricles to pump blood effectively. The main causes of cardiogenic shock are myocardial infarction, arrhythmia, cardiomyopathy and valvular lesions. Patients are often cold and clammy (due to peripheral vasoconstriction), hypotensive, tachycardic and pale. There may be evidence of right ventricular failure (distended neck veins) or left ventricular failure (shortness of breath from pulmonary oedema). An ischaemic event will be evidenced by ECG changes and a 12-hour troponin.

4. E – Class III hypovolaemic shock

Femoral fractures are often associated with significant blood loss. This man presents with tachycardia, hypotension and a low urine output that can be graded as class III hypovolaemic shock.

5. G – Neurogenic shock

Neurogenic shock occurs secondary to injury of the sympathetic nervous pathways. The resulting loss of vasomotor tone and failure of the heart rate to increase causes a profound hypotension that may be mistaken for hypovolaemia. Features of neurogenic shock include hypotension, bradycardia and warm extremities. Management is with the use of inotropes (such as noradrenaline and vasopressin, to increase peripheral vascular resistance) and atropine (to reverse bradycardia). Causes of neurogenic shock include spinal cord injury above the T5 level, spinal anaesthesia, hypoglycaemia and closed head injuries.

Neurogenic shock is different to spinal shock, which occurs after an acute spinal cord transection and involves the loss of all voluntary and reflex activity below the level of the injury. Patients present with hypotonic paralysis, areflexia, loss of sensation and bladder retention.

THEME 3: MANAGEMENT OF CHEST TRAUMA

1. A – Analgesia and respiratory support

A paradoxical movement of the chest wall with respiratory distress is characteristic of flail chest. In flail chest, a segment of the chest wall loses continuity with the remainder of the rib cage. It is often defined as when two or more consecutive ribs are broken in two or more places. The flail segment can be seen to push in on inspiration and push out on expiration. Flail chest is always associated with a degree of pulmonary contusion, so respiratory distress and hypoxia may be apparent, as well as the chest pain caused by the broken ribs. Management of flail chest is with respiratory support and adequate analgesia, such as an epidural or intercostal nerve block. Operative intervention is rarely required.

2. E – Chest drain insertion

This woman is haemodynamically stable but is in some respiratory distress. The unilateral findings of decreased air entry and dullness to percussion suggest that she has suffered a haemothorax. A haemothorax describes the accumulation of blood in the pleural cavity. A haemothorax has the potential to be significantly large, as each side of the thorax can hold 30% of the circulating blood volume. Large haemothoraces are accompanied by hypovolaemic shock (hypotension, tachycardia and peripheral vasoconstriction). A haemothorax requires treatment by inserting a wide-bore chest drain into the fifth intercostal space in the anterior axillary line (along with adequate fluid resuscitation). Large-bore IV access should be established before chest drain insertion. A massive haemothorax is defined when more than 1500 mL of blood is removed from the chest cavity on initial insertion of the chest drain. A thoracotomy is indicated if the immediate blood loss on drain insertion is >2000 mL or if there is a continuing loss of >200 mL/h.

3. J – Pericardiocentesis

Cardiac tamponade, defined as accumulation of fluid within the pericardium, is often caused by penetrating knife injuries. The chambers of the heart most often injured are the left and right ventricles. The diagnosis of cardiac tamponade is made by Beck's triad of hypotension (due to reduced stroke volume), a raised jugular venous pressure (impaired venous return to the heart) and muffled heart sounds (secondary to the effusion). Other signs of cardiac tamponade are pulsus paradoxus, where there is a significant drop in arterial blood pressure (>10 mmHg) on inspiration, and Kussmaul sign, when the jugular venous pressure elevates on inspiration. An electrocardiogram will display low-voltage QRS complexes. As the condition progresses, electromechanical dissociation cardiac arrest occurs.

Immediate treatment of cardiac tamponade is by pericardiocentesis. A cannula is inserted at the costal margin, just to the left of the xiphoid process, aiming towards the left shoulder tip. Even the removal of 15 mL of blood can provide temporary relief until an urgent thoracotomy can be performed. Complications of pericardiocentesis include pneumothorax, cardiac arrhythmias and cardiac damage.

Greek *xiphoeides* = 'sword-shaped'.

Claude Schaeffer Beck, American thoracic surgeon (1894–1971).

Adolf Kussmaul, German physician (1822–1902).

4. I – Needle thoracocentesis

This woman has the typical features of a tension pneumothorax: unilaterally decreased breath sounds, hyper-resonance to percussion, respiratory distress and tracheal deviation away from the affected side. A raised jugular venous pressure may also be seen. If a tension pneumothorax is suspected then management should be immediate without ordering a chest X-ray. A large-bore cannula is inserted in the second intercostal space in the mid-clavicular line of the affected side. A hissing sound should be audible on decompression of the chest. This is later followed by formal chest drain insertion.

5. B – Apply a three-sided occlusive dressing

This man has a chest wound that is resulting in a pneumothorax, as suggested by the respiratory distress, reduced breath sounds and hyper-resonance to percussion. The undisplaced trachea means that the pneumothorax is not under tension. Management of an open pneumothorax is initially by occluding the wound with a sterile dressing and taping down three sides only. The resulting 'flutter valve' allows air to leave the chest on expiration but prevents it being sucked into the chest on inspiration. Subsequent management is by chest drain insertion at a different site.

THEME 4: DIAGNOSIS OF ABDOMINAL PAIN

1. I – Pelvic inflammatory disease

Acute pelvic inflammatory disease (PID) is caused by ascending infection from the vagina or cervix causing inflammation of the upper tract. Common pathogens include *Chlamydia trachomatis* and *Neisseria gonorrhoea*. Presenting features include lower abdominal pain, deep dyspareunia (pain during intercourse), dysuria and a vaginal discharge. Some people also develop Fitz-Hugh-Curtis syndrome – a right upper quadrant pain caused by inflammation of the connective tissue around the liver by the pelvic infection. Any patient presenting with suspected PID should have a urinary β-hCG test to rule out pregnancy. A specimen needs to be taken to look for offending pathogens, but treatment with appropriate antibiotics is commenced immediately to reduce the risk of long-term damage. A typical antibiotic regimen includes 2 weeks of ofloxacin (anti-chlamydia and gonorrhoea) and metronidazole (anti-anaerobe and protozoa).

2. J – Perforated peptic ulcer

This woman has presented with peritonitis. With her history of osteoarthritis, this is likely to be due to a perforated peptic ulcer secondary to use of NSAIDs. Perforated peptic ulcers present with sudden-onset severe abdominal pain that is referred to the shoulders due to diaphragmatic irritation and is worse with movement. Patients may also complain of nausea, vomiting, haematemesis or melaena. Examination reveals a shocked patient (cold, sweating, shallow respirations) with a rigid abdomen and absent bowel sounds. A diagnosis can de made using an erect chest X-ray that shows air under the diaphragm (a highly sensitive test). Immediate treatment includes 'drip and suck' (fluids and NG insertion), analgesia, antibiotics and a proton pump inhibitor. Urgent operative repair of the ulcer can subsequently be performed if suitable. Other drugs that increase the risk of peptic ulcer include SSRIs and steroids.

3. F – Irritable bowel syndrome

Irritable bowel syndrome (IBS) usually affects young and middle-aged women. The diagnosis is based on the Rome II criteria as follows: abdominal discomfort lasting for at least 12 weeks of the last 12 months (not necessarily consecutively) that has two of the three following features: (1) relieved by defaecation; (2) associated with a change in frequency of stool; and (3) associated with a change in consistency of stool. Before diagnosing IBS, it is important to exclude a serious underlying cause for the symptoms.

4. C – Chronic pancreatitis

The recurrent episodes of pain with only a mildly raised amylase indicate pancreatitis of a chronic nature. Chronic pancreatitis is the gradual, irreversible destruction of the pancreas. Excess alcohol consumption is the most common cause, although it can also be caused by cystic fibrosis, hypercalcaemia and hyperlipidaemia. Clinical features include recurrent severe epigastric pain that is better on leaning forwards, steatorrhoea (due to pancreatic enzyme insufficiency), diabetes (exocrine insufficiency) and obstructive jaundice (swelling of the pancreas resulting in biliary obstruction). An abdominal X-ray may show pathognomonic calcification in the pancreas. A CT scan demonstrates a large irregular pancreas. Levels of amylase are normal or only mildly raised, due to the loss of ability of the damaged pancreas to synthesize it.

The diagnosis of chronic pancreatitis can be confirmed by measuring the faecal elastase content – elastase being a pancreatic enzyme that is excreted via faeces. A reduced faecal elastase indicated moderate or severe pancreatitis. Management of chronic pancreatitis includes removing causative factors, analgesia, a low-fat diet, oral pancreatic enzyme supplements and control of diabetes. Many patients are on long-term strong opioids because of the painful nature of the disease.

5. K – Subphrenic abscess

A subphrenic abscess is a localized collection of pus under the diaphragm that occurs 10–20 days after generalized peritonitis. Typical features are malaise, nausea, abdominal pain that radiates to the shoulder (referred pain from dermatomes C3 to C5), anorexia and a swinging pyrexia. A chest X-ray shows a fluid level under the diaphragm, elevation of the diaphragm and collapse of the lung base. The diagnosis is confirmed by CT, and management is with antibiotics and drainage (either percutaneously or surgically). Features of a pelvic abscess are similar, but localizing symptoms include diarrhoea, urinary frequency, rectal mucus discharge and a boggy mass palpable on rectal or vaginal exam.

THEME 5: HAND DISORDERS

1. D – Ganglion

A ganglion is the most common cystic swelling at the back of the wrist. They are benign and can occur around any joint. Surgical resection may be required if troublesome. Historically, the treatment involved hitting the cyst with a heavy book causing it to rupture and drain the fluid into the surrounding tissues. As the heaviest book in most homes was the bible, ganglions developed the nickname 'Gideon's disease' or 'bible bumps'.

Ganglion, from Greek *ganglio* = swelling or knot.

2. A – de Quervain tenovaginitis

In de Quervain tenovaginitis, the sheath of the extensor pollicis brevis and abductor pollicis longus tendons becomes inflamed and thickened. It is most common in middle-aged women. De Quervain tenovaginitis is characterized by pain over the radial styloid. Abduction of the thumb against resistance and passive ulnar deviation of the wrist or thumb causes pain (Finkelstein test). A fibrous nodule may be palpable along the course of the tendons. The cause of de Quervain tenovaginitis is unknown, but some cases may be due to overuse. Treatment is by rest and steroid injections, or by operative de-roofing of the tendon sheaths.

3. J – Trigger finger

Trigger finger (digital tenovaginitis stenosans) is caused by thickening and constriction of the mouth of the tendon sheath, which interferes with free movement of the contained flexor tendons. The affected tendon becomes swollen distal to the sheath constriction. This means that it is easy to flex the tendon (as the swollen nodule slides out of the tendon sheath) but difficult to extend the finger without help. The thickening of the sheath forms a palpable nodule at the base of the finger. Treatment is by incising the mouth of the fibrous flexor sheath longitudinally.

4. B – Dupuytren contracture

Dupuytren contracture is a progressive fibroplasia of the palmar facia that results in a flexion contracture of the fingers. It is most common in the ring and little fingers. Risk factors include male sex, a family history, diabetes mellitus, alcoholic cirrhosis, phenytoin use, trauma/manual labour, AIDS, Peyronie disease (idiopathic fibrosis of the corpus cavernosum) and Ledderhose disease (fibrosis of the plantar fascia, resulting in a similar deformity). On examination, the thickened palmar aponeurosis can be felt. Treatment is by excision of the thickened part of the aponeurosis.

5. I – Thenar space infection

The thenar space and the mid-palmar space are two compartments of the palm that lie between the flexor tendons and the metacarpals. The thenar space is located on the lateral half of the palm, and the mid-palmar space on the medial side. Infection of these spaces leads to gross swelling of the palm. Treatment is by antibiotics, elevation and splintage. If minimal response is seen, early incision and drainage is essential.

Paronychia is an infection between the side of the nail and the lateral pulp of the finger. The term 'whitlow' describes an infection of the fibrofatty pulp of the finger. Tendon sheath infections produce rapid swelling of the affected digit. The features of tendon sheath infections are summarized by Kanavel signs: (1) tenderness over the flexor sheath; (2) pain on passive extension; (3) flexed posture of the digit; and (4) fusiform swelling of the digit. Tendon sheath infections require urgent incision, drainage and washout with intravenous antibiotics.

Paronychia, Greek *para* = next to + *onyx* = nail.

Gamekeeper's thumb (or skier's thumb) is tearing of the ulnar collateral ligament of the thumb metacarpophalangeal joint. It is seen in gamekeepers who wring the necks of small animals (some may say they deserve it!) and in skiers who fall onto the extended thumb, forcing it into hyperabduction. Partial tears are treated by plaster splintage. Complete tears require operative intervention.

Mallet finger (or baseball finger) occurs when sudden passive flexion of a distal interphalangeal (DIP) joint (like a ball striking the tip of the finger) ruptures the extensor tendon at the point of its insertion into the base of the distal phalanx. The DIP joint rests in mid flexion and cannot be actively extended. Treatment is by splinting the affected finger with the DIP extended and the proximal interphalangeal (PIP) joint flexed, to allow the tendon to reattach.

Whitlow is an infection of the finger tip. There are two forms: herpetic and melanotic. Whitlow should not be confused with paronychia (see above to compare and contrast).

THEME 6: DIAGNOSIS OF BILIARY TRACT DISEASE

Gallstones, or cholelithiasis, are rare in children but their incidence increases with age. The adage of the typical sufferer being fat, fair, female, fertile, flatulent and forty+ is rarely representative. Gallstones are more common in women, people of Mediterranean descent and those who have a history of rapid weight loss (including those patients who have had gastric bypass or gastric banding procedures). Other risk factors are Crohn's disease, chronic liver disease, pregnancy and previous infections of the biliary tract. There are three main types of gallstone. Cholesterol stones are yellow and greasy to touch and are more likely to occur in people with high cholesterol levels, who will have bile that is saturated with these compounds. Cholesterol stones are radiolucent. Bile pigment stones, which constitute the minority of gallstones, are small, black, irregular, gritty stones made of calcium bilirubinate. Because of their calcium content, these stones are radio-opaque. They occur most commonly in people with haemolytic disease, as this results in a large production of bilirubin. Most gallstones are a mixture of bile pigment and cholesterol, made up of alternate layers of each.

1. D – Cholangiocarcinoma

Cholangiocarcinoma is an uncommon tumour affecting the common bile duct. Risk factors for the development of these tumours include ulcerative colitis, primary sclerosing cholangitis, bile duct stones and bile duct cysts. Cholangiocarcinomas are generally adenocarcinomas and commonly occur at the confluence of the right and left hepatic ducts (in which case they are called Klatskin's tumours). Patients present with painless progressive jaundice, dark urine and pale stools, epigastric pain, steatorrhoea, and weight loss. The tumours are slow-growing, but there is no curative treatment and prognosis is poor. Instead, palliative stenting of the common bile duct by ERCP or surgical bypass can be performed to improve the symptoms of biliary obstruction.

2. J – Mirizzi syndrome

Mirizzi syndrome describes the scenario where there is a stone within the gallbladder in Hartmann pouch that presses extrinsically on the common bile duct, resulting in obstruction and features of obstructive jaundice. In other words, in Mirizzi syndrome, there is jaundice with pale urine and dark stools, but no stone within the common bile duct. In some cases of Mirizzi syndrome, the gallstone erodes from Hartmann pouch into the bile duct, forming a fistula through which further stones can pass. It is important to recognize Mirizzi syndrome pre-operatively as it can lead to biliary injury, especially with laparoscopic surgery.

Pablo Luis Mirizzi, Argentine physician (1893–1964).

3. F – Chronic cholecystitis

Chronic cholecystitis (or gallbladder dyspepsia) is caused by repeated inflammation of the gallbladder by stones. The gallbladder eventually becomes fibrosed and thickened. The symptoms of chronic cholecystitis are non-specific but include upper abdominal pain that starts a few minutes after eating and lasts about an hour. The pain is worse after fatty foods. The diagnosis is made based on these features and the finding of gallstones on abdominal ultrasound. Treatment is with elective laparoscopic cholecystectomy.

4. K – Primary sclerosing cholangitis

Primary sclerosing cholangitis is an inflammatory condition characterized by chronic fibrosis of the intra- and extra-hepatic biliary tree. It is more likely to develop in people with ulcerative colitis, retroperitoneal fibrosis, or HIV infection. (Secondary sclerosing cholangitis can be due to bile duct stones or strictures.) Patients present with jaundice, intermittent fever, pruritus and right upper quadrant pain. An ERCP will show beading of the biliary tree, due to intermittent multiple structuring. Symptomatic treatment is with steroids but, as it is a progressive disease, definitive management requires a liver transplant. Average survival time without transplantation is between 10 and 12 years. Sclerosing cholangitis is a risk factor for developing cholangiocarcinoma.

5. B – Ascending cholangitis

Ascending cholangitis is an infection of the common bile duct (CBD) that may be secondary to an impacted bile duct stone but can be caused by any factor that results in biliary stasis (i.e. biliary stricture or malignancy). It can be a life-threatening illness. Bacterial infection typically ascends from the duodenum, but can spread haematogenously from the portal vein in rare cases. Patients present with Charcot's triad of symptoms: jaundice + right upper quadrant pain + fevers/rigors. The CBD becomes filled with pus, and drainage is required urgently along with antibiotics (e.g. cefuroxime and metronidazole). The common bile duct is normally 6–7 mm in diameter. A dilated CBD may indicate a distal obstruction. The woman in this scenario has a CBD of 9 mm, suggesting that a distal stone is causing biliary stasis, which, in turn, is resulting in the development of ascending cholangitis.

Jean-Marie Charcot, French neurologist (1825–1893).

THEME 7: INVESTIGATION OF UROLOGICAL DISEASE

1. C – CT scan

Haematuria is the cardinal sign of renal injury and may only appear hours after the offending trauma. Sudden profuse haematuria can occur between 3 days and 3 weeks after trauma when a clot becomes dislodged. Bleeding into the retroperitoneum may result in abdominal distension. Closed kidney injuries are described as one of four grades: grade 1 – subcapsular haematoma, grade 2 – laceration of the kidney, grade 3 – avulsion of one pole of the kidney, and grade 4 – avulsion of the kidney from the vascular pedicle.

This man has undergone a potentially dangerous trauma. Although he is stable, he requires investigation for the haematuria. A CT scan with contrast will highlight any disruption in the renal tract as well as any other intra-abdominal injury. If there are signs of progressive blood loss (tachycardia, low blood pressure) or an expanding loin mass, surgical exploration is indicated.

2. B – Bladder scan and urethral catheterization

The presentation of suprapubic pain, a suprapubic mass and the inability to micturate suggest a diagnosis of acute urinary retention. The three most common causes of acute retention are benign prostatic hyperplasia, prostate carcinoma and urethral stricture. In the emergency situation, retention can quickly be confirmed by bladder scanning. A urethral catheter is inserted to relieve the obstruction and prevent the development of obstructive uropathy. Should a residual volume be greater than 500 mL, renal function should be checked in case of hydronephrosis.

3. A – Anterograde urethrogram

Injury to the urethra can be classified as anterior or posterior. Anterior injuries affect the penile and bulbar urethra and occur following 'straddle' injuries or instrumentation of the tract. Posterior injuries (of the membranous urethra) occur after pelvic fractures. Urethral trauma presents with blood at the urethral meatus, an inability to micturate and a palpable bladder. Anterior urethral trauma may also produce butterfly bruising of the perineum. If urethral injury is suspected, an immediate anterograde urethrogram should be performed. This is done by inserting a catheter just inside the urethral meatus and then injecting water-soluble contrast. If this confirms urethral injury, a suprapubic catheter should be inserted.

4. D – Cystoscopy and retrograde ureteric stent

This man has hydronephrosis following impaction of a ureteric calculus in his only functioning renal tract. Calculi typically become lodged in one of three narrowings of the renal tract. These are the pelvi-ureteric junction, vesico-ureteric junction and the point at which the ureter enters the pelvis. This requires urgent intervention before he develops failure of his remaining kidney. Because he only has one kidney left, the best option would be cystoscopy with retrograde placement of a ureteric stent to relieve the obstruction (this is because percutaneous nephrostomy carries a risk of damaging the kidney).

Hydronephrosis is an aseptic dilatation of the kidney due to partial or complete obstruction of urine flow. Unilateral hydronephrosis can be due to tumour, stones, retroperitoneal fibrosis or instrumentation. Bilateral hydronephrosis is due to urethral obstruction, or arises when a cause of unilateral hydronephrosis occurs bilaterally. Hydronephrosis results in the inability of the kidney to excrete (resulting in post-renal renal failure) and pressure-related damage to the renal parenchyma.

5. H – Transrectal ultrasound and biopsy

This man presents with a raised prostate-specific antigen (PSA) and it is likely that he has a prostate malignancy. PSA is a proteolytic enzyme made by the prostate that helps liquefy semen so that sperm can swim freely. Levels are increased with prostate cancer, benign prostate hypertrophy, increasing age, urinary tract infections, urethral instrumentation and recent ejaculation. (Digital rectal exam does not raise serum PSA.) Normal PSA levels are <4.0 ng/mL, but the likelihood of prostate cancer increases with a raised PSA (20% if PSA is 4–10 ng/mL, 60% if PSA is 10–20 ng/mL and 90% if PSA > 20 ng/mL).

The diagnosis of prostate cancer is by transrectal ultrasound with biopsy. Multiple random biopsies are taken in an attempt to gain a representative sample of the prostate. Prostate cancer is graded according to the Gleason score. The Gleason score is the sum of two numbers. The first number represents the most common tumour pattern (1–5) seen among biopsies. The second number represents the second most common tumour pattern.

Donald Gleason, American pathologist (1920–2008).

THEME 8: LOWER GASTROINTESTINAL HAEMORRHAGE

1. B – Angiodysplasia

Angiodysplasia describes the presence of multiple small vascular malformations, usually dilated veins, in the colon. It is more common in the elderly. Although angiodysplasia can occur anywhere in the bowel, it occurs most frequently in the caecum and ascending colon. Angiodysplasia is usually asymptomatic, but some lesions can bleed, resulting in recurrent frank per rectum blood loss or iron deficiency anaemia from chronic blood loss. The diagnosis is made by colonoscopy. Lesions appear as dilated submucosal vessels, but they may easily be missed. An actively bleeding lesion of angiodysplasia can be detected by mesenteric angiography, as contrast leaks into the bowel lumen. Treatment is by diathermy of lesions. In some cases of continued bleeding when the offending lesions cannot be found, a total colectomy may be performed as life-saving treatment.

2. H – Infective colitis

The short history of bloody diarrhoea and diffuse abdominal pain with vomiting suggests a diagnosis of infective colitis. Blood-stained diarrhoea is more likely to be from a bacterial pathogen, such as *Campylobacter*, *Salmonella* or *Shigella*. Management is by rehydration, using either oral rehydration therapy or intravenous fluids if the patient is vomiting. A stool culture should be sent off, and unless this comes back negative, antidiarrhoeal agents such as loperamide should be withheld.

3. E – Diverticular disease

The long history of abdominal pain relieved by defecation and the lack of weight loss make a diagnosis of colorectal carcinoma less likely. A diverticulum is an outpouching of a hollow structure. Colonic diverticula are examples of false diverticula, i.e. their walls are made up only of the inner mucosal layer of the bowel. A true diverticulum involves all the layers of the wall from which it arises (e.g. Meckel diverticulum). Diverticulosis describes the presence of colonic diverticula. Diverticular disease is a term used if complications arise from diverticulosis (as in this scenario). Finally, diverticulitis specifically describes inflammation of the diverticula.

Colonic diverticula are most commonly found in the sigmoid and the descending colon. They are unusual in the under-40 age group, but 30% of the elderly populations of developed countries are found to have diverticulosis at autopsy. The pathogenesis of diverticulosis is as follows: there is hypertrophy of the muscle of the sigmoid colon, resulting in high intraluminal pressures. This leads to herniation of the mucosa at potential sites of weakness in the bowel wall corresponding to points of entry of blood vessels. The underlying aetiology of the initial large bowel hypertrophy is unknown, but it may be directly due to a chronic low-fibre diet. Complications of diverticulosis include diverticulitis, lower gastrointestinal haemorrhage from erosion of a blood vessel within a diverticulum, and obstruction/stenosis from chronic diverticular infection and fibrosis. The diagnosis of diverticulosis is made by flexible sigmoidoscopy. Barium enema shows the diverticular outpouchings with a signet ring appearance due to filling defects produced by pellets of faeces within the diverticula. In the acute phase of suspected diverticulitis, CT is the best investigation.

4. C – Colorectal cancer

In a man of this age presenting with altered bowel habit, with or without rectal bleeding, colorectal cancer must be excluded. Colorectal carcinoma (CRC) is the second most common malignancy in the UK and is more prevalent in females. Sixty percent of cases occur in the colon and 40% in the rectum, with the sigmoid colon being the most common site of colonic malignancy. The vast majority of CRC develops sporadically (i.e. there is no pattern of inheritance); however, risk factors include familial adenomatous polyposis (FAP) and hereditary non-polyposis colorectal cancer (HNPCC).

FAP is caused by an autosomal dominant mutation in the adenomatosis polyposis coli (APC) gene. Affected persons have multiple polyps in the colon and small intestine. Polyps first appear in adolescence and present with bleeding and diarrhoeal episodes. Malignant change within these polyps is inevitable, and usually occurs between 20 and 40 years of age. FAP accounts for 3% of cases of colon cancer. Individuals with FAP have hypertrophy of the retinal pigment layer.

HNPCC is an autosomal dominant disorder of DNA mismatch repair that accounts for 5% of cases of colon cancer (FAP 3%, 3 letters, HPNCC 5% 5 letters). The occurrence of colon cancer in three or more family members over two generations, with one under the age of 50, strongly suggests HNPCC (the 3-2-1 rule). This is known as the Amsterdam criteria. HNPCC is also associated with tumours of the ovary, uterus and stomach.

In the sporadic CRC pattern, two genetic abnormalities are seen propagating the adenoma-carcinoma sequence. 85% of these occur from chromosomal instability, the remaining 15% are from microsatellite instability.

Colon cancer can present differently, depending on the site of the tumour. Left-sided tumours can present with fresh bleeding and obstruction (because stools on the left are more solid). Right-sided tumours often present with iron deficiency anaemia due to chronic blood loss. They rarely cause obstruction. Diagnosis of tumours is by colonoscopy and biopsy. A barium enema will show a characteristic 'apple-core' lesion. The management of colorectal tumours is by appropriate resection and post-operative chemotherapy with 5-fluorouracil. If resection is not possible, a palliative colostomy can be performed to relieve obstruction.

5. D – Crohn's disease

The long history of right iliac fossa pain, a right iliac fossa mass and the passage of blood in a teenager should alert you to a diagnosis of Crohn's disease. Crohn's disease is a non-specific inflammatory disorder of the gastrointestinal tract that is characterized by full-thickness inflammation and non-caseating granulomas. This is in contrast to the superficial inflammation that occurs in ulcerative colitis. Crohn's disease can occur anywhere in the GI tract, from mouth to anus, and skip lesions occur. The mucosal ulceration along with the intermittent oedema that occurs in Crohn's disease results in a cobblestone appearance of the bowel. Forty percent of cases affect the terminal ileum.

Crohn's disease typically presents in young adults with abdominal pain and diarrhoea. A mass may be palpable in the right iliac fossa, and this represents the inflamed terminal ileum. Those with active disease may also have fevers, anorexia and weight loss. Mouth ulcers can also occur.

Perianal manifestations, such as the development of fissures, fistulae, skin tags and abscesses, are relatively common in Crohn's disease. Extra-intestinal manifestations of Crohn's disease include oxalate renal calculi, arthritis, erythema nodosum and pyoderma gangrenosum. Erythema nodosum is a panniculitis of the shins caused by an immune response to a variety of triggers. The cause for these red tender nodules can be remembered by the pneumonic SORE SHINS [Sarcoid, OCP, Ricketssia, Eponymous (Beçhets disease), Streptococci, Hansen's disease (leprosy), IBD, non-Hodgkin lymphoma, Sulphonamides]. Diagnosis of Crohn's disease is by endoscopy and biopsy. Small bowel enema in Crohn's disease demonstrates stricturing in the affected segments, resulting in a classical radiological appearance known as the string sign of Kantor.

Acute episodes of Crohn's disease are managed using an elemental diet and steroids. An elemental diet is a liquid preparation of amino acids, glucose and fatty acids. Milder symptoms can be treated with salicylate drugs, such as mesalazine. Immunosuppressants such as mesalazine and azathioprine can also reduce the frequency and severity of relapses. Surgery is reserved for chronic severe disease or recurrent disease. Surgery should aim to be as conservative as possible, since patients with Crohn's disease are at risk of requiring multiple resections and developing short bowel syndrome.

THEME 9: TUMOUR MARKERS

Tumour markers may be used in different settings. They are most effective, though, in establishing cancer recurrence and assessing response to therapy. They can be used as screening tools, but clinicians should be aware of their specificity and sensitivity.

1. D – CA 15-3

This woman has a breast tumour that may be accompanied by a rise in the tumour marker CA 15-3.

2. G – Carcinoembryonic antigen

Colorectal tumours are associated with the tumour marker carcinoembryonic antigen (CEA).

3. I – Prostate-specific antigen

The features of poor stream and terminal dribbling may be apparent with benign prostatic hypertrophy and prostate carcinoma. A digital rectal examination would be appropriate, along with measurement of serum PSA.

4. J – S-100

Malignant melanomas are associated with positive histological staining with S-100.

5. E – CA 19-9

Painless progressive jaundice and a palpable gallbladder indicate a tumour at the head of the pancreas. An appropriate tumour marker is CA 19-9, which has a sensitivity and specificity of 80–90% for pancreatic cancer.

Other examples of tumour markers include:

α-fetoprotein	→ hepatocellular carcinoma
CA 125	→ ovarian carcinoma
Neurone-specific enolase	→ small cell lung cancer
Placental alkaline phosphatase	→ ovarian carcinoma, testicular tumours
Acid phosphatases	→ prostatic carcinoma
β-hCG	→ choriocarcinoma, testicular tumours
Monoclonal IgG (paraprotein)	→ multiple myeloma
Calcitonin	→ medullary thyroid cancer
Thyroglobulin	→ thyroid tumours (follicular/papillary)

THEME 10: INVESTIGATION OF BREAST DISEASE

The risk of developing breast cancer doubles with each decade of life until the menopause, at which time it falls. In addition to age, risk factors include previous breast disease, family history and cancer in the other breast. The principal breast cancers include invasive ductal carcinoma, in-situ ductal carcinoma, invasive lobular carcinoma, in-situ lobular carcinoma and Paget disease.

1. H – No further investigation

Any breast lump should be investigated by triple assessment. This consists of clinical examination, imaging and tissue sampling. This woman has undergone all three. The findings of multiple cysts with fibrosis and epithelial hyperplasia, along with the clinical symptoms, strongly suggest a diagnosis of fibrocystic disease. Hence no further investigation is required.

2. I – Ultrasound scan

This young woman has a single breast lump that has only been examined. The next stage of triple assessment is imaging. In most cases, the primary mode of imaging is mammography, i.e. an X-ray of the breast. Women under the age of 35 years have breast tissue that is more dense, so mammography is not as reliable. It is for this reason that in women under 35 years an ultrasound scan is the first-line imaging technique.

3. F – Magnetic resonance imaging

In women who have breast implants, an MRI scan is the best mode of imaging.

4. C – Core biopsy

Fine-needle aspiration cytology in this woman yields dysplastic cells. We cannot be sure whether the dysplasia represents ductal carcinoma in situ or whether there has been invasion of the basement membrane. This is because aspiration cytology only shows specific cells, not their relation to the rest of the tissue. The only way to distinguish between carcinoma in situ and invasive carcinoma is by core biopsy (also known as a Trucut biopsy). The tissue core can then be sent for histology to confirm the presence or absence of invasive cancer.

5. B – Aspirate cytology

The management of breast cysts is by aspiration alone in most cases. You should be aware that a minority of breast cysts may contain a malignant focus within their walls. A blood-stained aspirate from a breast cyst may be an indicator of malignancy, so the sample should be sent for cytology to look for dysplasia.

THEME 11: PENILE CONDITIONS

1. G – Phimosis

The term 'phimosis' means non-retraction of the foreskin, and includes congenital non-retractile prepuce, non-retraction due to scarring and lichen sclerosis, a fibrosing condition of unknown aetiology where the tip of the foreskin becomes tight, white and fixed to the glans. Lichen sclerosis of the penis is also known as balanitis xerotica obliterans. In cases of phimosis not due to lichen sclerosis, the prepuce may balloon on micturation. In these cases, gentle retraction of the prepuce is advised and circumcision is not indicated. In balanitis xerotica obliterans, the narrowed prepuce may eventually lead to urinary obstruction, and circumcision is required.

Paraphimosis is caused by retraction of a tight foreskin over the glans. The foreskin then acts as a tight band, impeding venous outflow from the glans and resulting in oedema, making it more difficult to reduce the skin. The management of paraphimosis is by administering a local anaesthetic ring block to the glans, followed by simultaneous squeezing of the glans and reduction of the foreskin. After paraphimosis, formal circumcision should be done to prevent recurrence. The prepuce should be returned to cover the glans of the penis following urethral catheterization. Failure to do so can result in iatrogenic paraphimosis.

2. A – Circinate balanitis

The triad of urethritis, arthritis and iritis is characteristic of Reiter syndrome, now more commonly known as reactive arthritis. (Hans Reiter had an affiliation with the Nazi political party and his name has subsequently fallen out of favour.) It is caused by underlying sexually transmitted infections or gastroenteritis. Two other features that can occur with Reiter syndrome are circinate balanitis and keratoderma blennorrhagicum. Circinate balanitis describes an annular, erythematous reaction on the glans penis and occurs in 30% of men with Reiter syndrome. Keratoderma blennorrhagicum describes the presence of pustular, crusty, yellowy-brown papular lesions on the soles of the feet that are clinically and histologically indistinguishable from pustular psoriasis. It is seen in 15% of males with Reiter syndrome.

Hans Conrad Julius Reiter, German bacteriologist (1881–1969).

3. F – Peyronie disease

Peyronie disease is a condition of unknown aetiology characterized by progressive fibrosis of the tunica albuginea covering the corpus cavernosum of the penis. It occurs in 1% of men around the age of 50 years and is associated with Dupuytren contracture. Symptoms of Peyronie disease begin with pain on erection, followed by deviation of erection and a ventral curvature of the penis. Deformity can progress until sexual intercourse becomes impossible. Some cases, but not all, are caused by trauma to the penis. A variety of medical treatment options are available, none of which have strong evidence for their efficacy. Surgical options include incision/excision of the fibrotic plaque or graft placement. Complications include worsening of the curvature and penile shortening.

Francois de la Peyronie, French surgeon (1678–1747).

Guillaume Dupuytren, French physician (1777–1835).

4. H – Priapism

Priapism is a prolonged, painful erection that is not associated with sexual desire. Prolonged erection leads to hypoxia and ischaemia within the corpora of the penis, and pain begins after 3–4 hours. After 12 hours, interstitial oedema develops, and smooth muscle necrosis occurs after 24 hours. Priapism can result in erectile dysfunction, with the risk depending on the duration of erection (43% if <24 hours, 90% if >24 hours). Management can be conservative (exercise, ice), medical (oral terbutaline or intracavernosal phenylephrine) or surgical (vascular shunts).

There are many underlying causes of priapism, including haematological disorders (sickle cell disease), malignant infiltration by solid tumours, neurological conditions (e.g. stroke) and drugs (anti-hypertensives and drugs used for erectile dysfunction).

Priapism, from Greek *priapismos* = erection.

5. E – Penile cancer

Penile cancer presents with a persistent ulcer of the glans, which may be associated with a bloody or purulent discharge. Around 50% of patients have bilateral inguinal lymphadenopathy at the time of presentation – this may represent inguinal node spread or inflammation. Penile cancer is a squamous cell carcinoma that is more common in elderly men in developed countries and is invariably due to chronic irritation of the glans by retained smegma under the foreskin (men who have been circumcised do not develop this tumour).

Diagnosis is by biopsy of the ulcer. Management of penile tumours depends on the stage, but options include penis amputation (penectomy), with or without inguinal lymph node dissection. Unresectable disease is managed by palliative radiotherapy.

THEME 12: CUTANEOUS MALIGNANCIES

1. J – Superficial spreading malignant melanoma

Malignant melanoma is a malignant tumour of melanocytes and is the most lethal of skin tumours. It is most common in Caucasians living near the Equator and is twice as common in women. Risk factors include repeated UV exposure, previous malignant melanoma, multiple melanocytic naevi and having a large congenital naevus. Primary treatment is by surgical excision. Prognosis is related to tumour depth (Breslow score).

Superficial spreading malignant melanoma is the most common type of malignant melanoma. It occurs most often in younger females on the leg. The tumour is macular with an irregular edge and may itch or bleed.

2. F – Keratoacanthoma

A keratoacanthoma (or 'molluscum sebaceum') is a benign tumour of hair follicle cells. It occurs on sun-exposed sites (e.g. face and arms) and is more common in the elderly. Keratoacanthomas grow rapidly over 6–8 weeks and are characterized by a rolled edge with a central keratin plug that can fall out and leave a crater. Spontaneous resolution occurs, but takes several months and leaves a deep scar. Keratoacanthomas are usually excised, as there is a small risk of transformation to squamous cell carcinoma and to avoid the deep scar. Squamous cell carcinomas are different to keratoacanthomas in that they grow slowly, there is no central core and they gradually ulcerate.

Keratoacanthoma, from Greek *kerat* = horn + ***akantha*** = thorn; a thorn of horn!

3. E – Bowen disease

Bowen's disease (or squamous cell carcinoma in situ) is a premalignant intra-epideramal carcinoma with atypical keratinocytes characterized by a well-defined erythematous macule with slight crusting that may be mistaken for eczema. It typically occurs on the legs and trunks of older women. Previous exposure to arsenic (often found in tonics) can predispose to the condition. A small percentage of these can progress to squamous cell carcinoma. Treatment is by excision. Erythroplasia of Queyrat is Bowen disease of the glans penis. It appears as a red, velvety lesion.

John Templeton Bowen, American dermatologist (1857–1941).

Louis Queyrat, French dermatologist (1872–1933).

4. I – Squamous cell carcinoma

Squamous cell carcinoma (SCC) is a malignant tumour of keratinocytes that occurs in the over-50 population in sun-damaged sites. Predisposing factors for its development include X-ray exposure, smoking, human papillomavirus and a genetic susceptibility. SCCs typically have raised everted edges with a central scab. The proliferating keratinocytes can give the lesion a 'pearl-like' appearance. Management is by surgical excision, with lymph node dissection or radiotherapy if there is evidence of spread.

An actinic keratosis (also known as a solar keratosis) is a hyperkeratotic, yellow-brown crusty lesion that occurs on sun-damaged sites. Although these lesions are benign, they are premalignant to SCC. For this reason, actinic keratoses should be removed, for example by excision, shaving or cryotherapy.

5. G – Lentigo maligna melanoma

The original lesion that this woman has on her cheek is a lentigo maligna (or Hutchinson's malignant freckle) – a large irregular pigmented area that occurs most often in elderly people on sun-exposed skin. Lentigo maligna is associated with malignant transformation to melanoma (lentigo maligna melanoma). Thickening, darkening or ulceration within a lentigo maligna signals the onset of malignancy.

Lentigo, from Latin *lentigo* = lentil; the word was originally used to describe freckles.

Other forms of malignant melanoma include nodular, acral lentiginous and amelanotic types. Nodular melanomas present as thick, protruding, smooth, sharply defined lesions that grow in a vertical direction and may bleed and ulcerate. They are the most aggressive of all melanomas as they invade vertically from the outset (there is no in situ growth phase). Nodular melanomas may not be pigmented (amelanotic melanomas) and this is associated with a poorer prognosis, as lesions are not as noticeable. Acral lentiginous melanomas (or subungual melanomas) present as expanding pigmented lesions on the palms, soles and nail beds. This is the most common presentation in Afro-Caribbean people.

Sir Jonathan Hutchinson, English surgeon and pathologist (1828–1913).

THEME 13: MANAGEMENT OF ENDOCRINE DISEASE

1. G – Surgical resection and radiotherapy

The older woman who presents with dysphagia associated with a large, irregular hard mass probably has anaplastic carcinoma of the thyroid gland. This tumour has a poor prognosis despite surgery, chemotherapy or radiotherapy. However, in cases where there are symptomatic issues, such as dysphagia, palliative surgery and radiotherapy can be used to relieve the obstruction. Placement of a tracheostomy and/or gastrostomy may also be required to aid breathing and feeding.

2. B – Carbimazole

This young pregnant woman presents with thyrotoxicosis and ophthalmoplegia, features typical of Graves disease. The first-line treatment in the under-40 age group is carbimazole, a drug that inhibits the production of thyroid hormones. Iodine-131 should be avoided in women who are pregnant or who are around children, due to the risk of radioactivity-induced teratogenicity.

3. C – Desmopressin

Polyuria and polydipsia has many causes, but when no other symptoms are apparent, you should consider diabetes insipidus. Diabetes insipidus (DI) is characterized by the excretion of excessive quantities of dilute urine with thirst, and is mediated by a lack of active antidiuretic hormone (ADH). ADH is secreted by the posterior pituitary gland and has the function of increasing water reabsorption in the collecting ducts of the nephron. There are two types: cranial DI (which is due to a lack of ADH secretion from the pituitary) and nephrogenic DI (which results from a lack of response of the kidneys to circulating ADH). Causes of cranial DI include head injury (as in this patient), surgery, sarcoidosis and the DIDMOAD syndrome (characterized by diabetes insipidus, diabetes mellitus, optic atrophy and deafness). Nephrogenic DI can be due to metabolic abnormalities (hypokalaemia, hypercalcaemia), drugs (lithium, demeclocyline), genetic defects and heavy metal poisoning.

Patients with DI may pass up to 20 litres of water in a day. The diagnosis of DI is confirmed using the water deprivation test. The patient is deprived of water and the urine and plasma osmolalities are measured every 2 hours. If there is a raised plasma osmolality (>300 mOsm/kg) in the presence of urine that is not maximally concentrated (i.e. <660 mOsm/kg), then the patient has DI. At this point in the test, the patient is given an intramuscular dose of desmopressin (a synthetic analogue of ADH). If the patient now starts concentrating their urine, then they have cranial DI. If the urine osmolality remains <660 mOsm/kg then nephrogenic DI is confirmed.

The treatment of cranial DI is with desmopressin. Nephrogenic DI is improved by thiazide diuretics.

4. I – Total thyroidectomy and thyroxine

This patient has an enlarging asymptomatic thyroid lump with lymphadenopathy. It is most likely that she has a papillary thyroid cancer. Papillary thyroid cancer is the most common of all the thyroid cancers accounting for approximately 80% of cases. It spreads via the lymphatics and is managed by total thyroidectomy, followed by daily thyroxine to help prevent recurrence of the tumour. Five-year survival is around 95%.

5. D – Hydrocortisone and fludrocortisone

The features that this young girl has are typical of adrenal insufficiency. This, along with the recent meningococcal septicaemia, points to an underlying diagnosis of Waterhouse-Friderichsen syndrome. Waterhouse-Friderichsen syndrome is bilateral haemorrhage into the adrenal glands caused by meningococcal septicaemia. The management of adrenal insufficiency is by replacement of glucocorticoids (by hydrocortisone) and mineralocorticoids (by fludrocortisone).

Rupert Waterhouse, English physician (1873–1958).

Carl Friderichsen, Danish pediatrician (1886–1979).

THEME 14: EYE DISEASE

1. B – Anterior uveitis

The uvea is the vascular anterior part of the eye, made up of the iris and the ciliary body. Anterior uveitis (or iritis) presents with acute-onset eye pain, photophobia, blurred vision and lacrimation. On examination, you can expect to find circumcorneal redness, a small irregular pupil and decreased visual acuity. A layer of yellowish material may be seen in the anterior chamber of the eye (known as a hypopyon). Talbot's test is a useful clinical examination: the patient is asked to follow your finger with their eyes as you move it towards them. In anterior uveitis, the eye pain increases as the eyes converge and the pupils constrict. Anterior uveitis occurs in middle-aged and young adults and is associated with HLA-B27 joint problems (e.g. ankylosing spondylitis, psoriatic arthritis, Reiter syndrome and enteropathic arthritis), sarcoidosis and Behçet disease. Treatment is with prednisolone drops (to reduce inflammation) and atropine drops (to keep the pupils dilated and prevent adhesions from forming).

Hypopyon, from the Greek *hupo* = 'below' + *puon* = pus/

2. G – Episcleritis

Episcleritis describes inflammation of the episclera, a thin membrane that covers the sclera. Episcleritis presents with painless reddening of the eye. It is common with autoimmune conditions, such as rheumatoid arthritis (as in this scenario). On examination, dilated blood vessels will be seen only in the superficial layer of the sclera. When a cotton bud is placed against the eye, these vessels can be moved over the sclera. Steroid eye drops provide symptomatic relief and aid recovery.

Scleritis describes inflammation of the sclera, which is less common but more serious than episcleritis. Patients present with redness of the sclera (i.e. if you try moving the dilated vessels with a cotton bud, they won't budge), severe ocular pain and photophobia. Repeated episodes of scleritis can result in thinning of this membrane over time (scleromalacia). Scleromalacia is seen as a blue-tinged area in the sclera. This area is prone to perforation → scleromalacia perforans. All the changes described can occur with rheumatoid arthritis.

3. A – Acute closed-angle glaucoma

Acute glaucoma (also known as acute closed-angle glaucoma) is caused by a blockage of the drainage of aqueous humour from the anterior chamber of the eye via the canal of Schlemm. It occurs most often in middle to old age. Features of acute glaucoma are severe eye pain, nausea and vomiting, with poor vision. On examination, the eye will be firm and tender, the cornea hazy, and the pupil fixed, dilated and ovoid in shape. Acute glaucoma requires urgent ophthalmological referral. Immediate management is with pilocarpine drops (a beta-blocker that results in miosis and subsequently opens up the previously blocked drainage canal) and intravenous acetazolamide (which reduces the formation of aqueous humour to help relieve the pressure in the eye). Once the pressure has been relieved medically, a bilateral iridectomy is performed, where a piece of the iris is removed to allow free circulation of the aqueous humour.

4. C – Blepharitis

Blepharitis is a chronic inflammation of the eyelids, usually by staphylococcal infection or seborrhoeic dermatitis. Patients present with burning itchy eyes, which is worse in the morning. On examination, the eyes and eyelids appear inflamed. A superficial crust may be seen on the lid margins, along with a reduction in the number of eyelashes. Treatment is with saline bathing and topical fusidic acid.

5. D – Conjunctivitis

This woman has bacterial conjunctivitis of her eye. Conjunctivitis presents with reddening and inflammation of the eye, along with lacrimation, itching and burning. Conjunctivitis can be allergic, viral or bacterial. Viral conjunctivitis often results in a watery discharge. Bacterial conjunctivitis is associated with a purulent discharge and is commonly caused by *Staphylococcus* or *Streptococcus* genus. Many cases resolve spontaneously, but chloramphenicol eye drops hasten the response.

The term 'hyphaema' describes the presence of blood in the anterior chamber of the eye. It often results from blunt trauma to the orbit. The presence of hyphaema should be managed urgently, as further bleeding can increase intraocular pressure and compromise sight.

A sty is a painful abscess of an eyelash hair follicle. Treatment is by removal of the offending eyelash with topical fusidic acid. An ectropion is an eversion of the lower eyelid, causing eye irritation, excessive lacrimation and keratitis. It occurs in older people due to a laxity of the orbicularis muscle. An entropion is an inturning of the eyelid (again, usually the lower lid). It occurs in older people due to degeneration of the fascial attachments of the lower eyelid. Permanent repair of both ectropion and entropion is surgical.

THEME 15: PREOPERATIVE MORBIDITY

The American Society of Anesthesiologists (ASA) grading system is the most commonly used scale to predict preoperative morbidity irrespective of the surgery that the patient is about to undergo. Patients are assigned a preoperative grade according to the following scale:

Grade I	Normal, healthy individual (0.05% anaesthetic mortality)
Grade II	Mild systemic disease that does not limit activity (0.4% mortality)
Grade III	Severe systemic disease that limits activity but is not incapacitating (4.5% mortality)
Grade IV	Incapacitating systemic disease that is constantly life-threatening (25% mortality)
Grade V	Moribund, not expecting to survive over 24 hours with or without surgery (50% mortality)

In addition to the above grading scale, an 'E' suffix is used to denote an emergency operation.

1. C – ASA grade II

This man's IBD is 'controlled' by medications and therefore will not limit his activity; hence he is grade II.

2. C– ASA grade II

Again, the hypertension will not limit this woman's activity, but it still counts as mild systemic disease; hence she is grade II.

3. E – ASA grade III

This woman's asthma must limit her life somewhat if she has required multiple admissions for it. However, it is a disease with exacerbations and is not constantly life-threatening (and thus she is not grade IV).

4. G – ASA grade IV

Chronic renal failure requiring dialysis would count as constantly life-threatening because if this woman did not receive her treatment, she would die.

5. J – ASA grade VE

Having a ruptured abdominal aortic aneurysm is a life-threatening condition, and a patient with this would be described as moribund. As this man is about to have an emergency procedure, he would be given the ASA classification of grade VE.

The ASA grading system has been widely adopted due to the efficacy with which information about physical health and sickness can be described between anesthetists and surgeons. The system is, however, limited by its failure to include 'local' disease states. Conditions such as ischaemic heart disease have a significant impact on perioperative mortality but are not systemic diseases and are therefore not accounted for.

THEME 16: BONE TUMOURS

1. A – Chondrosarcoma

A chondrosarcoma is a slow-growing malignant tumour of the cartilage that affects middle-aged patients. X-rays show localized bone destruction with areas of calcification within the tumour. Treatment is by chemotherapy with wide local excision.

2. C – Ewing sarcoma

Ewing sarcoma is an extremely rare malignant tumour of the bone that is most common in the 5- to 15-year age range. It is a small cell carcinoma that most commonly occurs in the legs or pelvis. Patients present with a painful swelling and fever. X-ray shows a lytic lesion with a laminated periosteal reaction, known as 'onion skinning'. Treatment is by neoadjuvant chemotherapy and/or radiotherapy with surgical excision.

3. I – Osteosarcoma

Osteosarcomas are the second most common primary bone tumours after multiple myeloma. Osteosarcoma occurs most often in young adults, in which case it may be associated with a history of retinoblastoma, and in older people with Paget disease. Osteosarcomas present with a warm, painful swelling, usually around the knee. X-ray features are characteristic, showing cortical destruction, periosteal elevation (Codman triangle) and calcification within the tumour but outside the bone (sunray spicules). Diagnosis is confirmed by biopsy, and treatment is by neoadjuvant chemotherapy with radical surgery. Osteosarcomas are very malignant tumours, and blood-borne metastases develop early and spread to the lungs.

4. F – Osteoid osteoma

An osteoid osteoma is a benign, painful, self-limiting tumour of the bone that occurs in children and young adults. It presents with intense pain that is characteristically worse at night and is relieved by NSAIDs. Osteoid osteomas are caused by a nidus of osteoblasts that become trapped in the cortex of the bone. X-rays show a radiolucent nidus surrounded by a dense area of reactive bone.

5. I – Osteosarcoma

As mentioned above, osteosarcomas are associated with Paget disease of the bone.

Enchondromas are common benign bone lesions of cartilaginous origin. They develop from aberrant cartilage left within a bone and are usually found in the metaphysis. Enchondromas are usually asymptomatic and are found incidentally. X-rays show a well-demarcated calcifying lesion within the metaphysis. Enchondromas can be single or multiple (Ollier disease). Osteochondromas are the most common benign bone lesions and develop from aberrant cartilage that remains on the surface of the cortex, most often around the knee. They present as an asymptomatic swelling. Diaphyseal aclasis is an autosomal dominant condition characterized by the presence of multiple osteochondromas. Osteoclastomas (giant cell tumours) are benign tumours of osteoclasts that occur around the epiphysis and are most common in young adults. These tumours are osteolytic and are slowly progressive. Treatment is by excision.

Secondary bone tumours are far more common than primaries. The five solid tumours that most commonly metastasize to bone are, starting with the most frequent, breast (35%), bronchus (30%), prostate (10%), kidney (5%), and thyroid (2%). Metastases from prostate tumours tend to be osteosclerotic (increase bone density), while those originating from the other tumours are osteolytic. Multiple myeloma is the most common secondary bone tumour. It is characterized by monoclonal immunoglobulins on serum electrophoresis, excess plasma cells on bone marrow examination and lytic lesions on plain X-ray. Patients present with bone pain, bacterial infection (from hypogammaglobulinaemia) and symptoms associated with hypercalcaemia.

THEME 17: MANAGEMENT OF ARTERIAL DISEASE

1. C – Best medical therapy

This man has intermittent claudication. Initial management is conservative (healthy diet, regular exercise, appropriate weight loss and cessation of smoking) along with best medical therapy (e.g. anti-platelet, anti-hypertensive and cholesterol-lowering drugs, along with good diabetic control if relevant). Surgery would be indicated if there were severe symptoms, ulceration, gangrene or critical limb ischaemia.

2. D – Embolectomy

This man has acute limb ischaemia secondary to an embolism, probably from the atrial fibrillation. An acutely ischaemic limb is a surgical emergency and needs to be resolved within 6 hours to prevent irreversible necrosis. Initial management is with oxygen and intravenous fluids, analgesia and immediate anticoagulation (5000 units of IV heparin). The next stage is to restore arterial continuity.

With embolus-induced ischaemia, management would be with either thrombolysis or surgical embolectomy. Thrombolysis is appropriate if the ischaemia is acute-on-chronic, since this means that the limb is not too acutely ischaemic and will remain viable for a long enough time to allow clot dissolution thanks to the development of collaterals. In thrombolysis, a cannula is inserted into the distal extent of the thrombus and streptokinase or tissue plasminogen activator is infused. Clot dissolution may take several hours. Complications of thrombolysis include anaphylaxis and haemorrhage. Contraindications to thrombolysis include recent surgery, recent stroke and bleeding tendencies.

The patient in this scenario has had a recent stroke, so he is not a candidate for thrombolysis. Instead, he should have a surgical embolectomy. In this procedure, a catheter with a deflated balloon on it (Fogarty catheter) is passed distal to the embolus. The balloon is then inflated and the catheter pulled out, dragging the embolus with it.

3. G – Fasciotomy

This man has suffered a reperfusion injury following management of an acutely ischaemic limb. When arterial continuity is restored following a period of occlusion, high concentrations of metabolites, such as potassium, myoglobin and lactate, are released back into the circulation simultaneously. These cause increased endothelial permeability and local tissue swelling. Unrelieved swelling can cause occlusion of arterial flow and further ischaemia – compartment syndrome. (More systemically, reperfusion can cause rhabdomyolysis and renal failure.) Features of compartment syndrome include severe pain (which is often out of proportion to the clinical findings), especially on stretching the affected muscle group, and sensory loss. Loss of distal pulses is a late sign.

Compartment syndrome is confirmed by measuring the compartment pressures in the leg using a green needle connected to a pressure transducer. If the compartment pressure exceeds 30 mmHg, then surgical intervention is indicated in the form of an urgent fasciotomy to relieve the pressure and avoid permanent muscle necrosis.

4. A – Amputation

This patient has developed gangrene secondary to chronic peripheral vascular disease. The fact that he has ulceration shows that his vascular disease has affected the distal vessels. Arterial bypass is only suitable if there is good distal run-off, and is thus not an option in this patient. Amputation is required urgently to prevent spread of gangrene.

Indications for amputation are remembered using the three Ds: dying (e.g. gangrene); dangerous (e.g. tumour, severe infection); and damned nuisance (e.g. neurological damage). The most common indication for amputation in the UK is peripheral vascular disease.

5. E – Endarterectomy left side

This woman has suffered a transient ischaemic attack (TIA, defined as a focal neurological deficit lasting less than 24 hours). TIAs can present as contralateral motor deficits (facial weakness or limb weakness) or ipsilateral visual disturbance, such as amaurosis fugax (a transient sudden vision loss in one eye due to passage of an embolus through the retinal artery). It is important to investigate and manage TIAs, as they are a major risk factor for subsequent stroke.

TIAs are often caused by atherosclerotic emboli originating from the carotid arteries. Carotid Doppler ultrasound should be performed in patients suffering with TIAs to detect significant stenosis. Patients who

have had a TIA/amaurosis fugax/stroke in the last 6 months in the presence of a carotid stenosis >70% are at high risk of subsequent stroke (30%). This group of patients may benefit from a carotid endarterectomy (removal of the diseased intima) as stroke prophylaxis. In patients who have a stenosis of <70%, or who have an asymptomatic stenosis, endarterectomy is controversial, and this group is probably best managed with conservative and medical therapy.

The woman in this scenario has suffered right-sided facial weakness; hence the embolus would have originated from the left carotid artery. Since her stenosis is greater than 70%, a left carotid endarterectomy is indicated. If she had instead suffered a right-sided amaurosis fugax then a right carotid endarterectomy would be more suitable.

Amaurosis fugax, from Greek *amaurosis* = darkness + Latin *fugax* = fleeting.

Postoperatively, carotid endarterectomy patients must be managed cautiously, particularly if they have bilateral disease. The carotid body contains chemoreceptors that provide short-term feedback on arterial pO_2. In bilateral disease, there may be a lack of a normal ventilatory response to opioids, resulting in acute hypoxia and death.

Practice Paper 5: Questions

THEME 1: GLASGOW COMA SCALE

Options

A. 0
B. 3
C. 4
D. 5
E. 6
F. 7
G. 8
H. 9
I. 11
J. 13
K. 14
L. 15

For each of the following scenarios, select the most likely option. Each option may be used once, more than once or not at all.

1. A patient is brought to the emergency department following a road traffic accident. He is not opening his eyes or making any sounds. The patient flexes abnormally in response to pain.
2. You are called to see a 54-year-old man following a liver resection. He is making noises but no understandable words. His eyes open in response to pain and he withdraws appropriately from painful stimuli.
3. An 84-year-old woman presents with urinary frequency and dysuria. She is sitting up with her eyes open and is moving spontaneously. However, her speech is occasionally confused and muddled.
4. A 24-year-old intravenous drug user is brought to the emergency department with a suspected opiate overdose. He opens his eyes in response to pain but makes no sounds. He withdraws from painful stimuli.
5. You are paged to see a patient who is extremely unwell. By the time you arrive, the nursing staff are performing cardiopulmonary resuscitation.

THEME 2: DIAGNOSIS OF HERNIAS

Options

A. Direct inguinal
B. Epigastric
C. Exomphalos
D. Gastroschisis
E. Hiatus
F. Incisional
G. Indirect inguinal
H. Paraumbilical
I. Spigelian
J. Umbilical hernia of infants

For each of the following scenarios, select the most likely hernia. Each option may be used once, more than once or not at all.

1. A term baby is born with large amounts of visible intestine emerging from of his abdomen. The external gut is covered with a thin membrane.
2. A 34-year-old man presents with a lower midline mass that is 8 cm in size. He has a history of an emergency laparotomy for toxic megacolon secondary to ulcerative colitis. On examination, the mass is soft, non-tender and reducible.
3. A 64-year-old man presents with two groin lumps, one on each side. On examination, the lumps have a cough impulse and are reducible but do not extend into the scrotum.
4. A 42-year-old woman presents to the emergency department with colicky abdominal pain and an abdominal lump. On examination, the lump is in the midline just above the umbilicus and is tender to touch.
5. A 39-year-old man presents to the emergency department with a 'tearing' pain in his upper abdomen after trying to lift weights at home. On examination, you find a 2 cm lump at the site of the pain in the midline of the abdomen, halfway between the xiphisternum and the umbilicus.

THEME 3: MANAGEMENT OF UROLOGICAL DISEASE

Options

A. Analgesia alone
B. Cystoscopy
C. Extracorporeal shock wave lithotripsy
D. Intravenous antibiotics
E. Lithotripsy
F. Nephrectomy
G. Percutaneous nephrolithotomy
H. Percutaneous nephrostomy
I. Suprapubic catheterisation
J. Three-way catheter and irrigation

For each of the following scenarios, select the most appropriate management. Each option may be used once, more than once or not at all.

1. A 38-year-old woman presents with left-sided loin pain, fever and rigors. On examination, there is a palpable mass on the left side. Her pulse is 106/min and her blood pressure 104/64 mmHg. A KUB film done in the emergency department shows a 7 mm stone at the vesicoureteric junction.
2. A 56-year-old male who has a 3-day history of frank haematuria presents with sudden-onset suprapubic discomfort and an inability to pass urine.
3. A 32-year-old man presents to the emergency department with severe right loin pain that radiates to the groin. On examination, there is microscopic haematuria on dipstick but no other abnormality. A KUB X-ray confirms the presence of a 4 mm stone in the ureter.
4. A 54-year-old man presents with loin-to-groin pain. An intravenous urogram shows a 1 cm stone in the renal collecting system.
5. A 62-year-old man presents with a 3-month history of left loin pain. Examination yields no abnormality. A KUB X-ray demonstrates a staghorn calculus in the left renal collecting system. A DMSA (dimercaptosuccinic acid) scan shows a split function of 10% in the left kidney and 90% in the right.

THEME 4: DIAGNOSIS OF HEPATOMEGALY

Options

A. Alcoholic cirrhosis
B. Amoebic liver abscess
C. Biliary tract obstruction
D. Budd-Chiari syndrome
E. Haemochromatosis
F. Hepatocellular carcinoma
G. Metastatic disease of the liver
H. Polycystic disease
I. Pyogenic liver abscess
J. Riedel lobe

For each of the following presentations of hepatomegaly, select the most likely diagnosis. Each option may be used once, more than once or not at all.

1. A 16-year-old girl presents with a 1-week history of right lower quadrant pain, nausea and anorexia. In the last 24 hours, she has become more unwell, developing spiking fevers and rigors. On examination, she appears mildly jaundiced. Her liver is enlarged and tender to palpation.
2. A 36-year-old woman presents to her general practitioner with a long history of vague abdominal pain. She denies any other symptoms, but

she mentions that she was admitted to hospital last year with a bleed in her brain. On examination, there is massive, nodular hepatomegaly.

3. A 42-year-old man attends his general practice with a history of excessive thirst and urinary frequency. On examination, he appears to be tanned, although he denies going abroad over the winter months. The liver is palpable 4 cm below the costal margin.
4. A 39-year-old man from India presents with a 2-week history of aching abdominal pain and weight loss. His past medical history includes eczema and a fractured femur in a car crash 20 years ago for which he received a blood transfusion. On examination, his abdomen is tender in the right hypochondrium and is mildly distended with a fluid thrill. His liver is enlarged and nodular.
5. A 26-year-old woman presents with sudden-onset severe upper abdominal pain. She takes the oral contraceptive pill, but has no other medical history. On examination, she is slim but has a distended abdomen that is positive for shifting dullness. The liver is palpable three finger breadths below the costal margin.

THEME 5: DIAGNOSIS OF THE SWOLLEN LIMB

Options

A. Congestive cardiac failure
B. Elephantiasis
C. Hereditary angioedema
D. Klippel-Trénaunay syndrome
E. Lymphoedema praecox
F. Lymphoedema tarda
G. Milroy disease
H. Post-radiotherapy lymphoedema

For each of the following presentations, select the most appropriate diagnosis. Each option may be used once, more than once or not at all.

1. An 84-year-old woman presents with worsening shortness of breath on exertion and difficulty breathing on lying flat. On examination, she has bibasal crackles and pitting oedema in both ankles.
2. A 16-year-old girl is admitted to the emergency department following sudden-onset oedema of her face, lips and limbs, along with difficulty breathing and abdominal pain. On examination, her face and limbs are massively swollen and itchy. Her abdomen is soft and bowel sounds are audible.
3. A 34-year-old woman attends follow-up at breast clinic 6 months after management for a primary breast carcinoma. She mentions that her left arm is swollen. On examination, there is no neurological deficit and all her peripheral pulses are palpable.

4. A 1-month-old baby boy is brought to the general practitioner with swelling of both lower limbs. On examination, there appears to be oedema of both legs below the knee that is non-pitting and firm to the touch.
5. A 46-year-old man presents with worsening swelling of his legs bilaterally. On examination, his legs are very oedematous and firm, and the skin is thickened, hard and grey in colour.

THEME 6: EPONYMOUS FRACTURES AND CLASSIFICATIONS

Options

A. Barton fracture
B. Bennett fracture
C. Colles fracture
D. Galeazzi's fracture–dislocation
E. Garden fracture
F. Le Fort fracture
G. Monteggia fracture–dislocation
H. Rolando fracture
I. Salter–Harris fracture
J. Smith fracture
K. Weber fracture

For each of the following descriptions, select the correct eponymous name or classification. Each option may be used once, more than once or not at all.

1. A 65-year-old woman suffers a subcapital fracture of the femoral neck following a fall.
2. A 3-year-old child has a fracture of the distal radius involving the growth plate.
3. A 72-year-old woman presents with wrist pain following a fall onto an outstretched hand. An X-ray shows a fracture of the distal radius with intra-articular involvement.
4. An 8-year-old boy presents following a fall on the outstretched hand. An X-ray of the affected upper limb shows a fracture of the upper ulna with dislocation of the radial head.
5. A 45-year-old woman twists her ankle after falling over in the rain. An X-ray of the ankle shows a fracture of the fibula below the level of the malleoli.

THEME 7: INVESTIGATION OF ABDOMINAL PAIN

Options

A. Creatine kinase levels
B. CT scan
C. Erect chest X-ray
D. Faecal elastase
E. Laparoscopy

F. Mesenteric angiography
G. Serum amylase
H. Supine chest X-ray
I. Troponin
J. Urgent laparotomy

For each of the following people presenting with abdominal pain, select the next appropriate investigation. Each option may be used once, more than once or not at all.

1. A 54-year-old man presents with a 3-day history of left upper quadrant pain, which is worse on inspiration, malaise and fevers. He also complains of a cough productive of green sputum. Abdominal examination is unremarkable.
2. A 56-year-old sheep farmer presents to his general practitioner with a 2-month history of abdominal aches and worsening jaundice. He denies weight loss or any other symptoms. On examination, a smooth mass can be felt in the right upper quadrant. An abdominal X-ray shows flecks of calcification in the right upper quadrant, separate to the liver and gallbladder.
3. An 84-year-old woman is brought to the emergency department with a 6-hour history of severe, colicky, central abdominal pain. On arrival, she is pale and sweaty, with an irregularly irregular pulse of 125/min and a blood pressure of 105/68 mmHg. There is diffuse tenderness on abdominal examination, and per rectum exam reveals fresh blood.
4. A 44-year-old man presents with recurrent episodes of severe epigastric pain that radiates to his back and is improved on leaning forward. On examination, he is jaundiced, with guarding in the epigastrium. There is no evidence of bruising. Observations are stable. Routine bloods are sent off and the amylase returns at 132 IU/L.
5. A 62-year-old man presents with sudden-onset tight epigastric pain that radiates up to his neck. He is also nauseated and is sweating. On examination, the abdomen is soft and non-tender. Bowel sounds are present and a per rectum exam is unremarkable. The pain is only relieved by morphine.

THEME 8: NIPPLE DISCHARGE

Options

A. Breast cancer
B. Breast cyst
C. Duct ectasia
D. Fat necrosis
E. Fibroadenoma
F. Fibrocystic disease
G. Galactocele
H. Gynaecomastia
I. Intraductal papilloma

J. Lactating breast
K. Peau d'orange
L. Phyllodes tumour
M. Prolactinoma

For each of the following people presenting with nipple discharge, select the most likely diagnosis. Each option may be used once, more than once or not at all.

1. A 21-year-old woman presents with a 4-month history of unilateral, painless, blood-stained discharge from the left nipple. On examination, no lumps are palpable on either side and there is no axillary lymphadenopathy. Cytology of the discharge reveals no malignant cells.
2. A 32-year-old woman has had multiple visits to her general practitioner over the last 6 months complaining of early morning headaches unresponsive to analgesia. On this occasion, she also admits to having a milky discharge from both nipples. A β-hCG urine test is negative and she has not had any children before.
3. A 45-year-old smoker presents to her general practitioner with a 6-month history of pain and a cheesy discharge from her left nipple associated with some inflammation of the areola. A mass can be felt under the areola, but no other lumps were palpable.
4. A 28-year-old woman is referred to you by her general practitioner with a 7-month history of amenorrhoea. She also complains of a whitish discharge from her nipples bilaterally. Her body mass index is 42 and she has no neurological symptoms. Breast examination is otherwise normal. She is worried as her mother has recently been diagnosed with metastatic breast cancer.
5. A 50-year-old woman presents with a 4-month history of a firm 3 cm lump in her right breast, with associated nipple inversion, a bloody discharge and axillary lymphadenopathy. Fine-needle aspiration cytology was reported as C5.

THEME 9: SKIN LESIONS

Options

A. Cavernous haemangioma
B. Deep capillary naevus
C. Dercum's disease
D. Ganglion
E. Granuloma annulare
F. Kaposi sarcoma
G. Neurofibroma
H. Pyogenic granuloma
I. Sebaceous cyst
J. Seborrhoeic keratosis
K. Superficial capillary naevus

For each of the following people presenting with skin lesions, select the most likely diagnosis. Each option may be used once, more than once or not at all.

1. A 12-month-old boy is brought to the general practitioner by his parents with a red lesion on his forehead. This was not present at birth, but has been growing for 3 months. On examination, the lesion is 2 cm, bright red and well-defined. There are no other symptoms.
2. A 25-year-old man presents with a lesion on his left wrist. On examination, there is a 2 cm firm lesion on the dorsum of the wrist that is painless and not mobile. There is no neurological deficit in the upper limb.
3. A 7-year-old boy is admitted to the emergency department with a seizure. On examination, he has a well demarcated purple, flat lesion over his left cheek and forehead. His parents say that this has been present since birth.
4. An 84-year-old man goes to his general practitioner with multiple dark brown, flat nodules on his back. These lesions are well-demarcated and are rough and greasy to touch.
5. A 46-year-old woman presents with multiple painful lesions over her body. On examination, each of these lesions is soft and mobile and 2 cm in size. She has no other symptoms.

THEME 10: DIAGNOSIS OF ANORECTAL DISEASE

Options

A. Anal carcinoma
B. Anal fissure
C. Anal fistula
D. Condylomata acuminata
E. Condylomata lata
F. Haemorrhoids
G. Perianal abscess
H. Perianal haematoma
I. Proctalgia fugax
J. Rectal prolapse

For each of the following people presenting with rectal symptoms, select the most likely diagnosis. Each option may be used once, more than once or not at all.

1. A 62-year-old man presents with a 2-month history of pruritus ani and occasional fresh blood on the toilet paper. He denies pain on defaecation. On examination, there is evidence of ulceration at the anal margin.
2. A 28-year-old man presents with a long history of intermittent pain in the rectum. The pain tends to occur at night. He denies passing any blood or mucous per rectum. Examination is unremarkable.

3. A 46-year-old woman complains of a stinging pain that occurs on defecation. This has been occurring for over a month. Rectal examination is very painful and there is a skin tag at the anal verge.
4. A 39-year-old woman presents with sudden-onset anal pain that occurred while straining at the toilet. On examination, a smooth, dark lump can be seen at the anal verge.
5. A 32-year-old man presents with a long history of pruritus ani. On examination, large pink, confluent lesions are seen around the anus.

THEME 11: INTRAVENOUS FLUIDS

Options

A. 0.45% sodium chloride solution
B. 0.9% sodium chloride solution
C. 4% dextrose/0.18% sodium chloride solution
D. 5% dextrose solution
E. Dextran
F. Gelofusin
G. Hartmann solution
H. Human albumin solution
I. Mannitol

For each of the descriptions, select the most appropriate intravenous fluid. Each option may be used once, more than once or not at all.

1. A fluid that contains around 150 mmol of sodium per litre.
2. A crystalloid that contains 5 mmol of potassium per litre.
3. The fluid that should be given as initial resuscitation in the trauma patient according to the Advanced Trauma Life Support guidelines.
4. A fluid that helps relieve raised intracranial pressure.
5. A fluid that helps decrease the risk of venous thrombosis.

THEME 12: MANAGEMENT OF PAEDIATRIC SURGICAL CONDITIONS

Options

A. Abdominal ultrasound
B. Air enema insufflation
C. Broad spectrum antibiotics
D. Gastrograffin enema
E. Observation
F. Pyloromyotomy
G. Laparotomy

For each of the following presentations, select the best management plan. Each option may be used once, more than once or not at all.

1. A 7-month-old baby presents with a 2-day history of intermittent abdominal pain and crying episodes. On examination, there is a mass in the upper abdomen. The doctor notices that the baby has passed blood and mucus motions in his nappy.
2. A 3-week-old boy presents with a history of projectile vomiting that occurs a few minutes after every feed. There is no bile or blood in the vomit. His mother says that despite the vomiting, the baby is still hungry for feeds.
3. A 3-day-old baby presents with a distended abdomen and bile-stained vomit. He is known to have cystic fibrosis. On examination, there are no masses in the abdomen and the rectum is empty.
4. An 11-year-old boy presents with a 24-hour history of right iliac fossa pain. He has no other complaints apart from a cold that started last week. On examination, his temperature is 37.5°C and he has cervical lymphadenopathy. Routine blood tests show a white cell count of 4.7 × 109/L.
5. A 7-day-old infant who was born preterm presents with bile-stained vomiting, abdominal distension and bloody diarrhoea. He is tachycardic and tachypnoeic on examination. An abdominal X-ray shows distended bowel loops with some intramural air.

THEME 13: EAR DISEASE

Options

A. Acoustic neuroma
B. Acute suppurative otitis media
C. Cholesteatoma
D. Chronic middle ear effusion
E. Chronic suppurative otitis media
F. Ménière disease
G. Otitis externa
H. Otosclerosis
I. Wax

For each of the following presentations of ear disease, select the most likely diagnosis. Each option may be used once, more than once or not at all.

1. A 40-year-old woman presents with a 6-month history of worsening deafness and a ringing sound in her ears. She also complains of occasional dizzy spells where she feels the room spins around her.
2. A 22-year-old woman presents with a 12-month history of worsening deafness in her left ear, especially to lower-frequency sounds. There is no evidence of tinnitus or dizziness. On examination, the patient admits that a vibrating tuning fork is louder when placed on the mastoid process on the left side, rather than by the ear. Examination of the ear is otherwise normal. The woman's mother developed bilateral deafness in her 30s.

3. A 48-year-old man presents with a 3-month history of a foul-smelling flaky discharge from his right ear. He admits to gradually losing hearing in this ear. On examination, a perforation is seen at the superior border of the attic.
4. A 65-year-old woman presents with a long history of ringing and hearing loss in her left ear. More recently, she has developed a headache. On examination, you notice that she has a weakness of the left side of her face, with forehead sparing. When a vibrating tuning fork is placed in the centre of the patient's forehead, the sound is heard better in the right ear.
5. A 6-year-old boy presents with a 2-day history of right-sided ear pain and a runny nose. He is constantly tugging at his ear. Examination of the ear shows an inflamed, bulging tympanic membrane.

THEME 14: KNEE CONDITIONS

Options

A. Anterior cruciate injury
B. Baker cyst
C. Chondromalacia patellae
D. Medial meniscus tear
E. Osgood-Schlatter disease
F. Osteochondritis dissecans
G. Osteoarthritis
H. Patellar dislocation
I. Pellegrini-Stieda disease
J. Prepatellar bursitis
K. Rheumatoid arthritis

For each of the following people presenting with knee problems, select the most likely diagnosis. Each option may be used once, more than once or not at all.

1. A 16-year-old girl presents to her general practitioner with a 2-month history of pain in her left knee. The pain is localised to the front of the knee and is worse on climbing stairs. On examination, there is no obvious swelling or bruising of the knee.
2. A 22-year-old man presents with sudden-onset pain and swelling in his right knee that occurred while walking. He denies any trauma to the knee. The patient describes his knee 'locking' at the time, although this sensation is not present now.
3. A 52-year-old woman has a 12-month history of worsening pain and swelling in her right knee, for which she has been taking regular analgesia. On examination, you can feel crepitus and the range of movement of the knee is limited by pain. A significant valgus deformity can be seen on standing.

4. A 14-year-old boy complains of a long history of pain in his left knee that is worse after exercise. On examination, there is a tender lump over the tibial tuberosity but no evidence of swelling or pain in the joint lines.
5. A 58-year-old man presents with pain and swelling directly over both patellae. He has just started a new part-time job as a builder. On examination, there is no other abnormality of the knee joints.

THEME 15: DIAGNOSIS OF VASCULAR DISEASE

Options

A. Buerger disease
B. Chronic venous insufficiency
C. Deep vein thrombosis
D. Embolus
E. Intermittent claudication
F. Ruptured Baker cyst
G. Spinal stenosis
H. Subclavian steal syndrome
I. Superficial thrombophlebitis
J. Takayasu arteritis

For each of the following people presenting with vascular disease, select the most appropriate diagnosis. Each option may be used once, more than once or not at all.

1. A 25-year-old man presents with a 2-month history of pain in the left calf on walking. He is now experiencing a similar pain on the right side. He smokes 20 cigarettes a day but denies having hypertension, hypercholesterolaemia or diabetes. On examination, all the limbs are warm. Distal pulses are palpable in the upper limbs but not in the lower limbs.
2. A 62-year-old woman presents to the emergency department with a 2-hour history of severe pain in her right leg. On examination, the patient's heart rate is irregularly irregular. Her right leg is cold compared with the left and the distal pedal pulses are not palpable.
3. A 72-year-old woman presents with a sudden-onset pain in her right calf. She has a past history of severe pain in both knees, for which she uses a walking stick and takes regular diclofenac. On examination, the calf is swollen, warm and tender when compared with the other side. A Doppler ultrasound performed in the emergency department showed no clot.
4. A 45-year-old woman who is in hospital following an elective cholecystectomy complains of pain and redness around her cannula site. On examination, she is stable and distal pulses are palpable. A painful cord-like structure is felt under the skin just proximal to the cannula.
5. A 24-year-old woman presents following an episode of dizziness and syncope preceded by right arm pain. Just prior to the episode, she was hammering picture hooks at home. Her boyfriend witnessed the episode

and he said that there was no fitting, tongue biting or incontinence. On examination, she has a bony lump palpable in the right side of her neck. Vascular and neurological examinations demonstrate no abnormality.

THEME 16: INVESTIGATION OF DYSPHAGIA

Options

A. 24-hour lower oesophageal pH
B. Anti-cardiolipin antibody
C. Anti-centromere antibody
D. Biopsy
E. CT chest
F. Endoscopy
G. Full blood count
H. Manometry
I. Muscle biopsy
J. Serial X-rays
K. Tensilon test

For each of the following people presenting with dysphagia, select the next appropriate investigation. Each option may be used once, more than once or not at all.

1. A 37-year-old woman presents with dysphagia that is equally apparent with solids and liquids. She also complains of regurgitation of food, which usually occurs on lying flat. She otherwise feels well, but admits to losing 5 kg in weight over the past 3 months. A chest X-ray shows an air–fluid level behind the heart, a double right heart border and absence of the gastric air bubble.
2. A 60-year-old man presents with occasional retrosternal chest pain that is worse on bending and lying flat. The pain is not relieved by analgesia. He also experiences a night cough. An electrocardiogram shows no acute changes, and troponin levels after 12 hours are negative.
3. A 45-year-old woman presents with a 2-month history of lethargy, occasional blurred vision and difficulty swallowing that is worse at the end of the day. She has no pain on swallowing and denies any other symptoms. Examination is unremarkable.
4. A 38-year-old woman present to the general practitioner with a 2-month history of dysphagia and worsening shortness of breath on exertion. On examination, you notice that she has multiple telangiectasias on her face and tight skin around her fingers causing fixed flexion deformities.
5. A 6-year-old boy is brought to the emergency department with pain in his throat after swallowing a penny coin earlier in the day. An X-ray confirms the presence of a foreign body in the duodenum.

THEME 17: UPPER LIMB NERVE LESIONS

Options

A. Anterior interosseous nerve
B. Lower brachial plexus
C. Distal median nerve
D. Distal ulnar nerve
E. Posterior interosseous nerve
F. Proximal median nerve
G. Proximal ulnar nerve
H. Radial nerve
I. Upper brachial plexus

For each of the following people presenting with neurological problems, select the most likely nerve involved. Each option may be used once, more than once or not at all.

1. A 37-year-old man presents with an abnormal tingling sensation in his left hand that occurs at night. The sensation is worse in his thumb and is relieved by hanging his hand over the end of his bed. He is awaiting surgical treatment for acromegaly.
2. A 22-year-old man presents following a motorcycle accident. He has fractured his right femur and also complains of pain in his neck. On examination, his right arm is hanging by his side, is medially rotated and is extended at the elbow. There is a loss of sensation on the lateral side of the right arm and forearm.
3. A 67-year-old man attends the emergency department following a fall. On examination, there is bruising on the right upper arm and the man is unable to extend his metacarpals on the same side. There is loss of sensation over the lateral dorsal aspect of the hand.
4. A 45-year-old woman presents following a fall on her outstretched hand. She is complaining of pain in her forearm. On examination, she cannot extend her fingers and can only weakly extend her wrist. There is no sensory loss.
5. A 22-year-old man attends the emergency department following a brawl in a night club. He has sustained a deep laceration to his wrist, as well as many other superficial cuts to his upper limbs. He complains that his hand feels weak. On examination, he has lost sensation over his 4th and 5th digits, but not over the palm.

Practice Paper 5: Answers

THEME 1: GLASGOW COMA SCALE

The Glasgow Coma Scale (GCS) is a subjective way of assessing and recording a patient's consciousness. The scale comprises three components: eye, verbal and motor response. The grades of each are as follows (the score should be based on the patient's best response):

Best eye response (E)

4 Eyes open spontaneously
3 Eyes open to speech
2 Eyes open to pain
1 No eye opening

Best verbal response (V)

5 Coherent speech
4 Confused/disorientated speech
3 Inappropriate words without conversational exchange
2 Incomprehensible sounds
1 No verbal response

Best motor response (M)

6 Obeys commands
5 Localizes to pain
4 Withdraws from pain
3 Abnormal flexion in response to pain (decorticate response)
2 Abnormal extension in response to pain (decerebrate response)
1 No motor response

The maximum score is 15 (E4, V5, M6) and the minimum is 3 (E1, V1, M1).

The GCS was first published in 1974 by Graham Teasdale and Bryan Jennett, both professors of neurosurgery at the University of Glasgow. Note there is a modified version of the scale: a 14-point scale which omits 'abnormal flexion'. The modified scale is also in use, including at the founding unit in Glasgow.

An alternative scoring score is AVPU. AVPU describes four levels of consciousness: alert, verbally responsive, responds to pain, unresponsive.

1. D – 5

This man is not opening his eyes (E1) or making any sounds (V1). He flexes abnormally to pain (M3). GCS = 1 + 1 + 3 = 5.

2. G – 8

This man opens his eyes with pain (E2), is making noises but no words (V2) and withdraws from painful stimuli (M4). GCS = 2 + 2 + 4 = 8.

3. K – 14

This woman's eyes are open (E4) and she is moving spontaneously (M6). She is able to speak, but her speech is confused (V4). GCS = 4 + 4 + 6 = 14.

4. F – 7

This man's eyes are open with pain (E2), but he makes no sound (V1). He withdraws to pain (M4). GCS = 2 + 1 + 4 = 7.

5. B – 3

This patient is having cardiopulmonary resuscitation. As such, he will have no eye opening (E1), verbal output (V1) or motor response (M1). GCS = 1 + 1 + 1 = 3. Remember the lowest GCS is 3, not 0!

THEME 2: DIAGNOSIS OF HERNIAS

1. C – Exomphalos

Exomphalos is a congenital abdominal wall defect where the contents of the gut, such as the intestines and liver, lie outside the body, protruding through the umbilicus. These organs lie within a sac made of two membranes – the inner being peritoneum and the outer being the amniotic membrane. This sac is known as an omphalocele. Treatment is by operative closure.

Gastroschisis is a similar congenital condition where abdominal contents lie outside the body without the covering membrane. An umbilical hernia of infants describes an asymptomatic herniation through a weak umbilicus that develops early in life. It is more common in Afro-Caribbean babies and increases in size on crying. Most umbilical hernias resolve spontaneously in the first two years of life, but surgery is indicated if they persist beyond this.

Omphalocele, from Greek *omphalus* = navel + *cele* = hernia.

Gastroschisis, from Greek *gastro* = belly + *schisis* = a split.

2. F – Incisional

Incisional hernias occur through a defect in a scar from a previous operation. Predisposing factors include poor nutrition, obesity, steroids, a chronic cough, poor wound suture technique and infection of the original wound. The neck of such hernias is usually wide, so strangulation is rare. Treatment is by dissection and re-suturing of the layers of the abdominal wall, with or without mesh insertion. Recurrence rates are variable, but lower with mesh repair.

3. A – Direct inguinal

Direct inguinal hernias protrude straight out of the abdominal wall through a weakened area of the transversalis fascia without travelling down the inguinal canal. The anatomic distinction between direct and indirect inguinal hernias is by their position relative to the inferior epigastric arteries. Direct inguinal hernias are found medial to the inferior epigastric arteries and indirect inguinal hernias are lateral to them. Direct inguinal hernias pass through Hesselbach triangle, a landmark bounded by the rectus muscle medially, the inferior epigastric vessels laterally and the inguinal ligament inferiorly. It is difficult to distinguish between direct and indirect on examination alone unless the hernia protrudes into the scrotum. Inguinal-scrotal hernias are always indirect. This has little clinical significance though, as the surgical approach is the same in each.

Direct inguinal hernias are always acquired and are bilateral in 12% of cases. Risk factors include smoking, obesity, heavy lifting and damage to the ilioinguinal nerve (which contributes to the nerve supply of the anterior abdominal wall and can be damaged with incisions to the lower abdomen, such as those gaining access to the appendix). The neck of direct inguinal hernias is wide and thus rarely strangulates. Symptomatic direct hernias can be repaired electively. Irreducible inguinal hernias with a history of less than 4 weeks should be repaired promptly as there is a higher risk of strangulation within the first 3 months.

Franz Hesselbach, German surgeon and anatomist (1759–1816).

4. H – Paraumbilical

This woman has a paraumbilical hernia. In adults, herniation can occur through the linea alba just above and below the umbilicus. (The linea alba is a fibrous median line formed by the fusion of anterior and posterior walls of the rectus sheath.) Paraumbilical hernias are much more common in multiparous women, and as they become large, they have a tendency to sag. Strangulation is a common complication, as paraumbilical hernias have narrow necks.

Linea alba, from Latin *linea* = line + *alba* = white.

Rectus abdominis, from Latin *rectus* = straight + *abdominus* = abdomen.

5. B – Epigastric

Epigastric hernias often occur in middle-aged men following lifting. Herniation occurs through a defect in the linea alba, which runs between the umbilicus and xiphisternum, and begins as a small protrusion of extraperitoneal fat that gradually enlarges.

THEME 3: MANAGEMENT OF UROLOGICAL DISEASE

1. H – Percutaneous nephrostomy

This woman presents with an infected hydronephrosis secondary to an impacted ureteric calculus. An infected obstructed system should be drained immediately, with emergency placement of a percutaneous nephrostomy, as the risk of renal damage is high.

2. J – Three-way catheter and irrigation

This man has developed acute urinary retention following obstruction by a clot. Initial management is by insertion of a three-way catheter and bladder irrigation to wash out the blood and clots. Further investigation into the source of bleeding will be required.

3. A – Analgesia alone

This man presents with a 4 mm ureteric calculus. Stones less than 5 mm in size do not require admission, since most of these (80%) pass harmlessly without intervention. Stones 5 mm or more only have a 20% chance of passing spontaneously. Adequate analgesia is usually sufficient, and diclofenac, an ANSAID, is the drug of choice (particularly effective when given per rectum).

4. C – Extracorporeal shock wave lithotripsy

Extracorporeal shock wave lithotripsy (ESWL) uses a concentrated acoustic impulse to shatter calculi. It is indicated for use in renal and upper ureteric stones that are <2 cm. For larger stones, it is important to insert a ureteric stent with ESWL to prevent a column of stone fragments from obstructing the ureter (known as *steinstrasse* or stonestreet). Contraindications to ESWL include pregnancy, an aortic aneurysm and uncorrected coagulation disorders. Flexible ureteroscopy is used for stones in the lower and mid-ureter and for those of the upper ureter that are not adequately managed by ESWL.

Percutaneous nephrolithotomy (PCNL) involves first gaining access to the renal collecting system by inserting a nephroscope. This allows larger stones to be broken down more directly. PCNL is used for stones >2 cm, such as staghorn calculi, or stones >1 cm in the lower pole calyx, which have poorer clearance rates with ESWL.

5. F – Nephrectomy

This man has a staghorn calculus in his left collecting system, for which there are two possible routes of management, depending on the function of the left kidney. A DMSA (dimercaptosuccinic acid) scan is a nuclear imaging scan that can be used to determine the split function (or the relative efficiency) of each kidney. If the kidney affected by the large stone has good function then percutaneous nephrolithotomy can be performed. However, if an affected kidney contributes <15% split function then nephrectomy should be considered.

THEME 4: DIAGNOSIS OF HEPATOMEGALY

1. I – Pyogenic liver abscess

This girl has developed pyogenic liver abscesses, most likely from an initial appendix infection. Pyogenic liver abscess can be single or multiple, and arises from infection in the portal system (appendicitis, diverticulitis or pelvic infection) or biliary tree. Clinical features include insidious onset of fever and rigors, swinging pyrexia, a tender palpable liver, and jaundice. The diagnosis is made by blood cultures and imaging. The initial treatment of choice is antibiotics with percutaneous drainage of abscesses. If symptoms still fail to resolve, then surgery is required. The mortality rate of pyogenic liver abscesses is 30%.

Amoebic liver abscesses occur secondary to *Entamoeba histolytica* infection of the large intestine. *Entamoeba histolytica* is a protozoan infection that is transmitted via the faeco-oral route. Approximately 10% of the world's population are asymptomatic carriers. The amoeba proliferate in the liver and can destroy the tissue (as the name suggests) to form a sterile abscess. Features are non-specific and include malaise, pyrexia and weight loss. The abscess can be identified on ultrasound. Management is with metronidazole, with or without drainage of the abscess. The motile feeding form of the amoeba (the trophozoite) can also penetrate the diaphragm and form pulmonary abscesses.

Entamoeba histolytica, from Greek *histo* = tissue + *lysis* = break down.

2. H – Polycystic disease

Adult-onset polycystic disease is an autosomal dominant condition characterized by cyst formation. Cysts can occur in any organ, but most commonly occur in the kidneys and the liver. Although the liver is massive, it still functions normally (unlike polycystic kidneys, which can develop renal failure). There is an association between polycystic disease and berry aneurysms in the circle of Willis, which may result in a subarachnoid haemorrhage.

A Riedel lobe is a congenital downward projection of the right lobe of the liver. It is a recognized anatomical variation and the lobe functions normally. A Riedel lobe may be mistaken for hepatomegaly on examination.

3. E – Haemochromatosis

Haemochromatosis is an autosomal recessive disorder of increased dietary iron absorption. Most cases affect Irish males over 40 years of age. There is systemic iron deposition, for example in the liver (cirrhosis), pancreas (diabetes), heart (cardiac failure), joints (arthropathy), testicles (impotence) and skin (tanned appearance). The diagnosis is confirmed by liver biopsy, which shows iron deposition with liver fibrosis and cirrhosis. Treatment is by weekly venesection of 500 mL until blood ferritin is normal. The main cause of death in haemochromatosis is hepatocellular carcinoma (below). Surgical treatment is reserved for end-stage liver disease and severe arthritis.

4. F – Hepatocellular carcinoma

Hepatocellular carcinoma is more common in areas where chronic hepatitis infection is prevalent. It is possible that the man in this scenario had transmitted hepatitis from his previous blood transfusion. Hepatocellular carcinoma usually occurs against a background of cirrhosis (e.g. due to hepatitis, excess alcohol ingestion or haemochromatosis). Another risk factor is aflatoxin, a metabolite of the fungus *Aspergillus flavus*. *Aspergillus* can contaminate nuts, grain and rice, and is a particularly significant problem in Africa south of the Sahara desert, where *Aspergillus* is found on up to 40% of screened foods. Patients present with jaundice, ascites and nodular hepatomegaly. The tumour marker α-fetoprotein is raised and imaging confirms the presence of tumours. Treatment is by liver resection, or transplant if the tumour is large.

5. D – Budd-Chiari syndrome

Budd-Chiari syndrome describes hepatic venous outflow obstruction. Risk factors include polycythaemia, thrombophilias, contraceptive pill use and malignancy. The syndrome presents with a classic triad of abdominal pain + ascites + hepatomegaly, although a high degree of clinical suspicion is required. The diagnosis of Budd-Chiari syndrome is made by Doppler ultrasound, which shows obliteration of hepatic vein flow and reversal of flow in the hepatic portal vein. Treatment is with thrombolysis or anticoagulation, but 70% of cases die within the year.

George Budd, English physician (1808–1882).

Hans Chiari, German pathologist (1851–1916).

THEME 5: DIAGNOSIS OF THE SWOLLEN LIMB

Lymphoedema is an accumulation of tissue fluid within the extracellular compartment due to a failure in the lymphatic system. Most cases (80%) occur in the lower limbs. Lymphoedema should be contrasted with oedema, which is an accumulation of tissue fluid in the absence of a lymphatic abnormality. Lymphoedema is a cause of non-pitting oedema. Another cause of non-pitting oedema of the lower limbs may be seen in Graves disease. It is known as pretibial myxoedema.

1. A – Congestive cardiac failure

Heart failure occurs when the heart cannot maintain adequate output. It is most commonly caused by hypertension, ischaemic heart disease and valvular disease. There is poor left ventricular function, which results in poor right ventricular function and congestion of fluid within the venous system. Features of heart failure include dyspnoea, orthopnoea, paroxysmal nocturnal dyspnoea, pulmonary oedema (inspiratory crepitations) and pitting oedema of the lower limbs. A diagnosis of heart failure is made by demonstrating poor left ventricular function on echocardiogram. Renal failure and hepatic insufficiency can also lead to lower limb oedema through a mechanism of either insufficient plasma protein production from the liver or protein loss from the kidney.

2. C – Hereditary angioedema

Hereditary angioedema is a rare and potentially fatal autosomal dominant deficiency of the C1-esterase inhibitor. The C1-esterase inhibitor acts as a mediator of complement proteins of the immune system, and a lack of this protein allows the complement system to go unchecked, with an accumulation of vasoactive inflammatory mediators. This can result in intermittent itchy swelling of the face, lips, pharynx and limbs along with abdominal pain, vomiting and diarrhoea. There is often no identifiable trigger for attacks of hereditary angioedema. Acute attacks are treated with intravenous C1-esterase inhibitor concentrate. Long-term management with anabolic steroids (e.g. danazol) help promote synthesis of C1-esterase inhibitor.

3. H – Post-radiotherapy lymphoedema

This woman, who has previously been managed for breast cancer, has lymphoedema. Treatment for breast cancer can involve axillary lymph node dissection and radiotherapy, both of which increase the risk of developing secondary lymphoedema. Radiotherapy results in lymph node fibrosis, which causes obstruction of lymph vessels. Malignant infiltration can also result in lymphoedema, so tumour recurrence should be considered in patients presenting years after radiotherapy. Patients should avoid having blood pressure measured and venipuncture from the affected side to reduce the risk of lymphoedema.

4. G – Milroy disease

Primary lymphoedema is more common in females and in those with a family history. It is classified according to the age of onset: congenital (Milroy disease is inherited autosomal dominant congenital lymphoedema, caused by a failure of lymph vessels to develop *in utero*); lymphoedema praecox (presents under 35 years); and lymphoedema tarda (presents over 35 years). Isotope lymphography, where a radioactive tracer is injected subcutaneously into the foot and its progress monitored, can be performed. A delayed transit time confirms the diagnosis. Management options for primary lymphoedema include compression, elevation, aggressive antibiotic therapy for infections and debulking surgery (indicated when conservative treatment has failed).

William Forsyth Milroy, American physician (1855–1942).

5. B – Elephantiasis

Elephantiasis (or lymphatic filariasis) is a cause of secondary lymphoedema. Elephantiasis is characterized by thickening of the skin and subcutaneous tissues, often of the legs and genitals. It is caused by infection and obstruction of lymph vessels by the parasite *Wuchereria bancrofti* in tropical countries. The infection is transmitted by mosquito bites.

Elephantiasis, from Greek *elephantas* = elephant; describing the appearance of the limbs in the affected patient.

THEME 6: EPONYMOUS FRACTURES AND CLASSIFICATIONS

1. E – Garden fracture

Fractures of the femoral neck are within the joint capsule. Such fractures are at risk of disrupting the blood supply to the femoral head, with subsequent avascular necrosis. Intracapsular fractures of the proximal femur are graded using the Garden classification:

Garden I	Impacted, stable fracture
Garden II	Complete but undisplaced fracture
Garden III	Partially displaced fracture
Garden IV	Completely displaced fracture

The blood supply is most likely to be disrupted in Garden III and IV fractures.

2. I – Salter–Harris fracture

The Salter–Harris classification describes fractures that involve the growth plate in children. The classification can be remembered using the initials SALTeR:

I	Slipped	Fracture across the physis with no other fragment
II	Above	Fracture across the physis with a metaphyseal fragment
III	Lower	Fracture across the physis with an epiphyseal fragment
IV	Through	Fracture through the physis with metaphyseal and epiphyseal fragments
V	Rammed	Crush injury to the physis

Remember that the metaphysis is the area of bone on the inside of the physis (growth plate) and the epiphysis is the outermost part of the bone.

3. A – Barton fracture

There are three eponymous fractures related to the distal radius. The most common is Colles fracture – a fracture of the distal 2.5 cm of the radius with dorsal and radial displacement of the distal fragment (leading to the classic 'dinner fork' deformity). A distal fracture of the radius that extends to involve the joint (i.e. intra-articular) is known as Barton fracture. Smith fracture is an extra-articular fracture of the distal radius that results in the opposite deformity to Colles fracture, i.e. volar (palmar) displacement of the distal fragment.

Abraham Colles, Irish surgeon and anatomist (1773–1843).
John Rhea Barton, American orthopaedic surgeon (1794–1871).
Robert William Smith, Irish surgeon (1807–1873).

4. G – Monteggia fracture-dislocation

Monteggia fracture-dislocation is caused by a fall with forced pronation of the forearm. It consists of a proximal ulna fracture with associated dislocation of the radial head. Galeazzi fracture-dislocation is a fracture of

the radial shaft, at the junction of its middle and lower thirds, with dislocation of the distal ulna. If you see a forearm fracture on an X-ray, you should always look for an associated dislocation.

Giovanni Monteggia, Italian surgeon (1762–1815).

Ricardo Galeazzi, Italian surgeon (1866–1952).

5. K – Weber fracture

Fractures of the distal fibula are classified using the Weber system as follows:

Type A	Fractures below the level of the tibial plafond
Type B	Fractures at the level of the tibial plafond (50% associated risk of disruption of anterior syndesmosis)
Type C	Fractures above the level of the tibial plafond

The more proximal the fracture is, the higher the risk of syndesmotic injury and instability. The tibial plafond is the lower flat border of the tibia. (Plafond, from French *plat* = flat + *fond* = base.)

A Bennett's fracture is a non-comminuted intra-articular fracture-dislocation occurring at the base of the first metacarpal. A Rolando fracture is a comminuted intra-articular fracture of the base of the first metacarpal. Le Fort fractures are fractures involving the mid-facial bones.

THEME 7: INVESTIGATION OF ABDOMINAL PAIN

1. H – Supine chest X-ray

The history of pain and a productive cough could be suggestive of lower lobe pneumonia with pain radiating to the abdomen. A chest X-ray would help confirm this diagnosis. It is important to consider the medical causes of abdominal pain, for example myocardial infarction, diabetic ketoacidosis, hypercalcaemia, uraemia, porphyria, vasculitis and sickle cell disease.

2. B – CT scan

Reaching the diagnosis here is difficult. In essence, this man has non-specific symptoms and a mass in the right upper quadrant. To delineate this mass better, the next investigation would be an ultrasound or CT scan (and only CT is on the option list). The diagnosis that ties this vague presentation is a hydatid liver cyst. Hydatid liver disease is most common in sheep-rearing communities and is caused by infection by the parasite *Echinococcus granulosus,* transmitted to humans by the excrement of dogs that eat sheep offal. The parasite penetrates the portal system to infest the liver and create a calcified cyst. Many cases are asymptomatic (90%), and cysts are found incidentally at postmortem. Symptoms can arise from the cyst compressing local structures. Occasionally, cysts can become infected or rupture, causing an allergic reaction which can potentially result in death. Should cystic fluid spill into the abdomen, further daughter cysts will also form. Hydatid disease is associated with a raised eosinophil count. The best way to image the cyst is by CT scan. If cysts are fully calcified, they can be left alone. The antiparasitic albendazole may shrink or kill the cyst, but larger lesions need surgical intervention. Intraoperatively, the cyst is exposed and some of the cystic fluid is aspirated. Saline or ethanol is then instilled into the cyst and left for 30 mins to ensure the parasite is dead before the entire cyst is then excised.

3. F – Mesenteric angiography

This woman has mesenteric vascular occlusion (mesenteric ischaemia). Mesenteric ischaemia describes acute occlusion of the mesenteric artery, which provides the blood supply to the gut. This can be by a thrombus, valve vegetation, a clot from atrial fibrillation (this scenario) or a paradoxical embolus that passes through a patent foramen ovale into the systemic circulation. The clinical features include acute colic, rectal bleeding and shock in an older patient. A high clinical suspicion is needed to diagnose mesenteric ischaemia. Immediate management is with blood resuscitation followed by an urgent mesenteric angiogram. This should be performed to confirm the diagnosis and find out if occlusion is due to a thrombus or an embolus. An embolus is managed by embolectomy and a thrombus is treated with an aorto-mesenteric bypass. Following this, any necrotic bowel should be resected. If the whole mesenteric supply is affected (small bowel and right colon) then the condition is fatal, unless there is revascularization from a saphenous vein conduit. Although not on the list of options here, a lactate would form part of the initial investigations (as a marker of intestinal ischaemia).

4. D – Faecal elastase

This man presents with features typical of chronic pancreatitis. A faecal elastase determination helps with diagnosis. Elastase is a pancreatic enzyme that is excreted via faeces. Reduced concentrations in the stools suggest moderate or severe chronic pancreatitis.

5. I – Troponin

Another medical cause of abdominal pain! A myocardial infarction may present with upper abdominal pain as opposed to chest pain. The radiation to the neck, sweating and nausea are common with ischaemic cardiac presentations. An ECG may show ST changes indicative of ischaemia, and a raised troponin after 12 hours would confirm the diagnosis.

THEME 8: NIPPLE DISCHARGE

1. I – Intraductal papilloma

Intraductal papillomas are benign localized areas of epithelial proliferation within large mammary ducts that are associated with an increased risk of developing invasive breast carcinoma. Patients present with a unilateral serous or serosanguineous (serous + blood) nipple discharge. On examination, a small lump may be palpable under the nipple. Mammography may be normal (or ultrasound if age ≤35 years). Expressed discharge normally shows epithelial cells and erythrocytes. Treatment is by excision of the affected duct (microdochectomy), due to the risk of developing malignancy.

2. M – Prolactinoma

The negative β-hCG test in this question confirms that the patient is not pregnant. As she has no children, we know that she is not breast-feeding. This is therefore an example of galactorrhoea – lactation in the absence of pregnancy or breast-feeding. The history of early morning headaches is typical of an intracranial space-occupying lesion. The most fitting diagnosis is therefore a prolactinoma.

Prolactin is a hormone secreted by the anterior pituitary gland. It stimulates the mammary glands to secrete milk. High levels of prolactin interfere with menstruation. A prolactinoma is a benign adenoma of the pituitary that secretes large amounts of prolactin. This results in galactorrhoea, irregular menses, subfertility and a decreased libido, as well as symptoms of an intracranial space-occupying lesion (e.g. early morning headaches, worse with coughing/straining). Other endocrine dysfunction may also be apparent secondary to compression of the pituitary.

3. C – Duct ectasia

In duct ectasia, the mammary ducts dilate and fill with a stagnant green-brown 'cheesy' secretion. This fluid may discharge from the nipple and irritate the surrounding areolar skin ('periductal mastitis'). Fibrosis of the duct eventually occurs, leading to nipple retraction. This condition is much more common in smokers. On examination, a subareolar mass (the dilated, filled ducts) may be palpable. Management is by stopping smoking and surgical excision of the major ducts (Hadfield procedure).

4. J – Lactating breast

This woman is morbidly obese (i.e. with a body mass index >40). She has a normal breast examination, despite the lactation. Considering the long history of amenorrhoea with the milky discharge, it is likely that this woman is pregnant but has not realized it. The fact that her mother has breast cancer is of no relevance. By contrast, galactorrhoea is the expression of milky discharge in the absence of pregnancy or lactation.

5. A – Breast cancer

This woman has breast cancer. Carcinoma of the breast often presents with a firm, irregular lump that may be attached to the overlying skin or to the pectoralis major muscle underneath. Other presenting features include nipple inversion, axillary lymphadenopathy, blood-stained nipple discharge and skin changes (Paget disease, peau d'orange).

Fine-needle aspiration cytology results are graded as follows:

- **C1** Inadequate sample
- **C2** Benign cells
- **C3** Equivocal, probably benign
- **C4** Suspicious, probably malignant
- **C5** Malignant cells (as in this case)

THEME 9: SKIN LESIONS

1. A – Cavernous haemangioma

A cavernous haemangioma (or strawberry naevus) is a condition that appears in the first months of life as a bright red lesion on the face or trunk that grows rapidly. Occasionally these lesions bleed or ulcerate. Cavernous haemangiomas eventually regress and disappear spontaneously, so intervention is only required if lesions persist beyond a few years of age. In such cases, yellow pulsed-dye laser followed by surgical excision can be organized. Cavernous haemangiomas may rarely be associated with thrombocytopenia and haemolytic anaemia secondary to trapping and destruction of platelets and erythrocytes within the lesions. This is known as Kasabach-Merritt syndrome.

Haig Kasabach, American paediatrician (1898–1943).
Katherine Merritt, American paediatrician (1886–1986).

2. D – Ganglion

A ganglion is a benign, tense, cystic swelling, often at the back of the wrist, that occurs due to degeneration of the fibrous tissue surrounding the joints. Ganglia are most common in young female adults. They are usually painless and asymptomatic, although they may occasionally press on adjacent nerves (ulnar and median nerves). Asymptomatic ganglia do not require treatment, and many spontaneously resolve. Lasting cure is by excision (aspiration is simpler, but 50% will recur). The traditional method of curing ganglia by striking them with a large Bible is no longer recommended. There is no convincing evidence for its effectiveness and it tends to do more harm than good!

3. B – Deep capillary naevus

A deep capillary naevus (or port-wine stain) is a malformation of the capillaries in the deep and superficial dermis. It is a congenital malformation that can occur anywhere in the body, but is most often found unilaterally on the face, neck or upper trunk. The area can become raised and thickened over time due to the proliferation of vascular and connective tissue. Occasionally, a port-wine stain is associated with seizures, mental retardation and eye abnormalities (glaucoma and optic atrophy) due to underlying cranial malformations. This is known as Sturge-Weber syndrome and is usually associated with a port-wine stain in the distribution of the ophthalmic or maxillary division of the trigeminal nerve.

Trigeminal, from Latin *tri* = three + *gemini* = twins, which together means 'triplets'. The trigeminal nerve has three divisions.

A superficial capillary naevus (also known as a salmon patch) is a small, flat, pink patch of skin with a poorly defined border. It is commonly found on the forehead (angel's kiss) or on the nape of the neck (stork mark). Most superficial naevi disappear in the first year of life.

William Allen Sturge, English physician (1850–1919).

Frederick Parkes Weber, English physician (1863–1962).

4. J – Seborrhoeic keratosis

Seborrhoeic keratoses (or basal cell papillomas) are common pigmented benign tumours of basal keratinocytes that often occur in large numbers on the face and trunk of elderly people. They are dark, rough and greasy and have a 'stuck-on' appearance with a well-defined edge. These lesions have no malignant potential, but may be removed by excision, curettage, cautery or cryotherapy if the patient wishes.

5. C – Dercum disease

This woman's lesions are lipomas – soft, mobile lesions composed of fatty tissue, which are usually painless. However, the presence of multiple painful lipomas is known as Dercum disease (or adiposis dolora). This occurs most commonly in obese middle-aged women and may be accompanied by headaches, amenorrhoea and reduced sweating. Simple lipomas can be removed by excision for cosmetic reasons.

Francis Xavier Dercum, American neurologist (1856–1931).

THEME 10: DIAGNOSIS OF ANORECTAL DISEASE

1. A – Anal carcinoma

Anal carcinomas are most often of the squamous cell type and are thought to arise from human papillomavirus (HPV) infection (types 16 and 18). Risk factors include the practice of anal sex and a history of genital warts. These tumours present after 50 years of age with bleeding, itching, pain and ulceration around the anus, often with associated inguinal lymphadenopathy. Anal carcinoma can be classified as anal margin or anal canal tumours depending on whether the cancer occurs above or below the dentate line. Small anal margin tumours (<2 cm) are managed by local resection, but most patients receive combination chemoradiotherapy as a first-line intervention. Anal canal cancers have a poorer prognosis, as they tend to be more locally invasive.

2. I – Proctalgia fugax

Proctalgia fugax is a benign condition that affects young, anxious men. It is characterized by brief attacks of rectal pain that usually occur at night and are unrelated to defecation. Management involves excluding organic disease, reassurance, analgesia and topical smooth muscle relaxants (e.g. GTN cream).

Proctalgia fugax, from Greek *proktos* = anus + *algos* = pain + *fugax* = fleeting.

3. B – Anal fissure

An anal fissure is a longitudinal tear at the anal margin that usually occurs after passing a constipated stool. Tears usually occur at the posterior margin, and multiple fissures may occur with Crohn's disease. Anal fissures can occur at the anterior margin in women, usually associated with giving birth. Patients present with a stinging pain that can last up to 2 hours following defaecation. This may be associated with small amounts of fresh bleeding and pruritus. On examination, the anal sphincter is in spasm and there may be a sentinel pile protruding from the anus (this represents a torn tag of the anal epithelium). Small anal fissures heal spontaneously, but more significant ones can be treated with nitrites or diltiazem cream, which relax the anal sphincter and allow the fissure to heal. Patients should also be advised of a high fibre diet. Chronic recurring fissures may need excision.

4. H – Perianal haematoma

A perianal haematoma (also known as a thrombosed external pile) is produced by thrombosis in the inferior rectal venous plexus. This plexus is covered by squamous epithelium with a somatic nerve supply, so thrombosis is very painful. Patients present with acute-onset anal pain while straining. Examination reveals a tense, smooth, dark blue, cherry-sized lump at the anal verge. In acute cases, management is by evacuation of the haematoma; otherwise rest and analgesia are appropriate.

5. D – Condylomata acuminata

This patient has features of anal warts. Anal warts are caused by human papillomavirus (HPV-6 and -11) and are spread by anal intercourse. Warts are often asymptomatic, but may present with itching, discharge or bleeding. On examination, pink and grey lesions may be seen around the anus and perineum. If these lesions are large and coalesce, they are known as condylomata acuminata.

Condylomata lata are large, fleshy, white lesions that occur in the genital region with secondary syphilis. They can be difficult to distinguish from condylomata acuminata, so, if you put this down, give yourself the mark!

Condylomata acuminata, from Latin *condylomata* = knuckles + *acuminatum* = pointed.

Condylomata lata, from Latin *lata* = broad.

THEME 11: INTRAVENOUS FLUIDS

1. B – 0.9% sodium chloride solution

Normal saline (or 0.9% sodium chloride solution) contains 154 mmol of sodium ions and 154 mmol of chloride ions. A 0.45% sodium chloride solution contains 77 mmol of each. Dextrose saline (4% dextrose/0.18% sodium chloride solution) contains 30 mmol of both sodium and chloride.

2. G – Hartmann solution

Hartmann solution is made up of 131 mmol/L sodium, 5 mmol/L potassium, 29 mmol/L bicarbonate, 111 mmol/L chloride and 2 mmol/L calcium. The other crystalloids in the list do not contain any potassium.

3. G – Hartmann solution

Hartmann solution is suggested by the Advanced Trauma Life Support guidelines to be the fluid of choice in the initial resuscitation of the trauma patient.

4. I – Mannitol

Mannitol is a plant-derived sugar alcohol. It is used clinically as an osmotic diuretic, especially to reduce an acutely raised intracranial pressure. Its use is controversial and awaiting a Cochrane review. Mannitol is also used as a sweetener and a mild laxative.

5. E – Dextran

Dextran is a complex, branched polysaccharide that is made up of glucose molecules. Dextran solutions are used in head and neck microsurgery to decrease the risk of vascular thrombosis. They do this by reducing erythrocyte aggregation and by inhibiting von Willebrand factor. Due to their potentially harmful side effects, such as anaphylaxis, acute renal failure and pulmonary oedema, there is debate as to whether dextrans should continue to be used for this purpose.

The decision on which intravenous fluid is most appropriate can be controversial. A recent Cochrane review (Perel et al. 2013) found that there was no evidence to support the use of colloids over crystalloids in the critically ill or injured, and that colloids may actually increase the risk of death.

NICE have recently released a new guideline titled Intravenous Fluid Therapy. It recommends that for resuscitation, a crystalloid that contains 130–154 mmol of sodium be used (i.e. Hartmann solution or 0.9% normal saline) with a 500 mL bolus given over 15 min. For maintenance, patients should receive 25–30 mL/kg/day of water, 1 mmol/kg/day of sodium, chloride, potassium and 50–100g of glucose to reduce starvation ketosis.

Perel P *et al.* Colloids versus crystalloids for fluid resuscitation in critically ill patients. *Cochrane Database Syst Rev* 2013: CD000567.

THEME 12: MANAGEMENT OF PAEDIATRIC SURGICAL CONDITIONS

1. B – Air enema insufflation

Intussusception is the invagination of proximal bowel into a distal segment, causing obstruction of blood flow to the inner bowel. It most commonly involves the terminal ileum passing into the caecum via the ileocaecal valve. Intussusception is most common in boys aged 6–9 months. Babies present with severe colicky pain and vomiting. During episodes, the child is pale and draws his or her legs up. A sausage-shaped mass may be palpable in the right upper quadrant. The passage of blood and mucus per rectum (redcurrant jelly stools) is a late sign. Management is by resuscitation followed by reduction of the intussusception by a rectal air enema. If this is ineffective (25% of cases), then operative reduction is required.

2. F – Pyloromyotomy

The presentation of non-bile-stained projectile vomiting soon after feeds in a hungry baby is indicative of pyloric stenosis. Pyloric stenosis is hypertrophy of the circular muscle of the pylorus causing gastric outflow obstruction. It presents in the first few weeks of life and most commonly affects first-born males. Apart from projectile vomiting, affected babies may be constipated and lose weight. A characteristic hypochloraemic, hypokalaemic metabolic alkalosis results from vomiting stomach acid. Pyloric stenosis is diagnosed by giving the baby a 'test feed': when the baby is given milk, visible gastric peristalsis may be seen over the epigastrium, and the pylorus is felt as an olive-shaped mass in the upper abdomen. If the diagnosis is in doubt, an ultrasound scan can be performed. After initial rehydration, management is by Ramstedt pyloromyotomy (where the muscle of the pylorus is cut longitudinally down to the mucosa). The baby can tolerate milk feeds a few hours after the operation.

3. D – Gastrograffin enema

This baby is known to have cystic fibrosis. A known complication of cystic fibrosis in neonates is meconium ileus (occurring in 15%), where a thick meconium plug causes intestinal obstruction. Affected babies will present with bile-stained vomiting and abdominal distension, and there will be no record of passage of meconium. In uncomplicated cases, a gastrograffin enema may help dislodge the meconium with its detergent and osmotic effects. If this fails then laparotomy is required.

4. E – Observation

The normal white cell count, the history of a recent cold and the presence of cervical lymphadenopathy make it more likely that this boy has mesenteric adenitis rather than acute appendicitis. Mesenteric adenitis describes inflammation of the mesenteric lymph nodes that occurs following an upper respiratory tract viral infection. It presents with features similar to acute appendicitis, and therefore it is important to get a detailed history and look for cervical lymphadenopathy. Mesenteric adenitis is a self-limiting condition, and if suspected, management should initially be conservative to avoid unnecessary laparotomy. Appendicitis is a clinical diagnosis and a period of observation with serial examinations can be very helpful. Should there be clinical deterioration, appendicitis becomes the more likely diagnosis and a laparoscopy +/– appendicectomy is indicated.

5. C – Broad-spectrum antibiotics

Necrotizing enterocolitis is a serious illness that affects preterm infants, especially those who are milk-fed. There is ischaemia of the bowel and infection by bowel organisms. Babies present with bile-stained vomiting, bloody diarrhoea and abdominal distension. This is rapidly followed by shock. Abdominal X-ray shows dilated bowel loops and thickening of the bowel wall with intramural air. Treatment is by parenteral nutrition and broad-spectrum antibiotics to cover both aerobes and anaerobes.

THEME 13: EAR DISEASE

1. F – Ménière disease

Ménière disease is an inner ear condition of unknown aetiology that is characterized by the 3 Ds: deafness (progressive sensorineural deafness), din (persistent tinnitus) and dizziness (intermittent rotational vertigo lasting a few hours). It is most common in those between 20 and 50 years, and a quarter of cases are bilateral.

Prosper Ménière, French physician (1799–1862).

2. H – Otosclerosis

This woman is going deaf in her left ear. The examining doctor has performed the Rinne test. In this investigation, a vibrating tuning fork of 512 Hz (an octave above 'middle C' for those of you of a musical ilk) is placed initially on the mastoid process (bone conduction), and then next to the ear (air conduction). The patient is then asked which sound was loudest. In the normal ear, air conduction (AC) is better than bone conduction (BC) – this is known as a positive Rinne test. In the woman in this scenario, BC is better than AC – a negative Rinne test, which, with left-sided deafness, is associated with a conductive hearing loss. Conductive hearing loss is a failure of conduction of sound waves through the middle ear. Conversely, sensorineural hearing loss is a failure of transmission of nerve impulses from the inner ear, via the vestibulocochlear nerve (cranial nerve VIII), to the brain. Of the available options, conductive unilateral hearing loss with a normal ear examination is most likely to be otosclerosis.

Otosclerosis is an autosomal dominant disorder characterized by abnormal bone formation around the stapes in the ear, resulting in conduction deafness. It usually occurs in young female adults. Deafness is progressive and usually begins with low frequencies. Patients can often hear better in noisy surroundings (paracusis). Treatment is by stapedotomy (replacement of the abnormal stapes with a prosthesis).

Otosclerosis, from the Greek *oto* = ear + *skleros* = hard; 'hardening of the ear'.

Heinrich Adolf Rinne, German ENT surgeon (1819–1868).

3. C – Cholesteatoma

A cholesteatoma is a chronic destructive infection of the middle ear that usually follows a previous chronic otitis media. Patients complain of a long history of foul-smelling, white, flaky discharge from the ear, that consists of stratified squamous keratinized epithelium. Other features include progressive deafness and vertigo. On examination, perforation of the attic (the bony wall of the middle ear) may be seen, along with a cholesteatoma cyst (a central mass of keratin debris in the middle ear). Cholesteatomas gradually eat into the surrounding tissue (e.g. dura mater and facial nerve) and bone (e.g. mastoid process), causing further complications, so treatment is essential. Lesions are removed by suction under microscopic view. Cholesteatomas may contain cholesterol.

Cholesterol, from Greek *chole* = bile + *steat* = fat; 'growth containing bile fats'.

4. A – Acoustic neuroma

The clinical test used by the examiner in this scenario is the Weber test. In this test, a vibrating 512 Hz tuning fork is placed in the middle of the patient's forehead. The patient is asked to report in which ear the sound is loudest. In conductive deafness, the sound is heard louder in the deafer ear. In sensorineural deafness, the sound is heard louder in the better ear. This woman is deaf in her left ear and Weber's test is louder in her right ear (the better one); therefore she has unilateral sensorineural deafness. In all cases of unilateral sensorineural deafness, an acoustic neuroma must be ruled out.

An acoustic neuroma is a benign tumour of the superior vestibular nerve in the internal auditory meatus or cerebellopontine angle. It presents with progressive sensorineural hearing loss with features of a raised intracranial pressure (morning headache that is worse with coughing and straining). Acoustic neuromas may impinge upon the trigeminal nerve (→ loss of corneal sensation) or the facial nerve (→ lower motor neurone facial nerve palsy). The diagnosis of acoustic neuroma is best made by MRI.

Acoustic, from Greek *akoustikos* = to hear.

Ernst Heinrich Weber, German physiologist and psychologist (1795–1878).

5. B – Acute suppurative otitis media

Middle ear infections can be acute or chronic. Acute otitis media describes acute infection of the middle canal, which most commonly occurs in young children following an upper respiratory tract infection. Common causes include *Streptococcus pneumoniae, Haemophilus influenzae* and *Moraxella catarrhalis*. Children present with ear pain and conductive deafness. On examination, the tympanic membrane is red, dull and bulging, due to the buildup of pus. If the tympanic membrane perforates, the pain settles and purulent, blood-stained fluid will be seen discharging from the ear. Management of acute suppurative otitis media is with antibiotics (e.g. penicillin).

If acute otitis media fails to heal, then the infection will continue with a persistent discharge and further damage to middle ear structures. This is known as chronic suppurative otitis media. Other complications of acute otitis media include acute mastoiditis (infection of the mastoid), meningitis and brain abscess development.

A chronic middle ear effusion ('glue ear') is a relatively common finding in children. There is accumulation of non-suppurative fluid in the middle ear resulting in reversible conductive deafness. Affected children may suffer behavioural change and impaired cognitive development due to chronic deafness. On examination, a dull tympanic membrane is seen in the absence of inflammation. Most cases of glue ear resolve spontaneously within 3 months. If symptoms persist beyond this, management is by grommet insertion.

Otitis externa is diffuse inflammation of the skin lining the external auditory meatus, often bacterial or fungal in origin. Features include outer ear irritation, scanty discharge and pain that is worse with jaw movement. It is most common in people with a narrow, tortuous ear canal and in patients who have traumatized the skin of the outer ear (e.g. by a towel or cotton buds). Note that the tympanic membrane remains intact in otitis externa.

Ear wax (cerumen) is produced by the ceruminous glands of the outer meatus and migrates laterally. Wax can be impacted in the ear by cotton buds and can result in deafness and irritation. Management is by ear syringing.

Cerumen, from Latin *cera* = wax + *albumen* = white.

THEME 14: KNEE CONDITIONS

1. C – Chondromalacia patellae

In chondromalacia patellae, the cartilage of the articular surface of the patella becomes roughened. The pain is caused by friction between the damaged area and the femoral condyle, hence its alternative name 'patellofemoral pain syndrome'. Chondromalacia patellae presents in teenage girls with an aching pain behind the kneecap that is exacerbated by climbing and descending stairs. X-rays show no abnormality. Should analgesia and physiotherapy not help, patients may require arthroscopy +/– chondroplasty.

Chondromalacia patella, from Greek *khondros* = cartilage + *malakos* = soft.

2. F – Osteochondritis dissecans

Osteochondritis dissecans is characterized by local ischaemic necrosis of a segment of the articular surface of a bone and its overlying cartilage. There is eventual separation of the fragment, resulting in an intra-articular loose body. The knee is the most common site for osteochondritis dissecans, especially the medial condyle of the femur.

Dissecans, from Latin *dissect* = to separate.

If the intra-articular loose body becomes trapped in the joint, the patient experiences sudden 'locking' of the knee associated with severe pain and swelling (as in this scenario). Loose bodies in the knee can often be seen with radiography and are usually found in the suprapatellar pouch (they are occasionally palpable here). Management is by removal of the loose body using arthroscopy.

3. G – Osteoarthritis

This woman has osteoarthritis, characterized by chronic knee pain with crepitus and a restriction of movement. The knee is the most common joint to be affected by osteoarthritis. In chronic cases, a valgus deformity is seen. (By contrast, in rheumatoid arthritis of the knee, a varus deformity is typical.) An X-ray of the joint may show typical features of osteoarthritis: narrowing of the joint space, subchondral sclerosis, bone cysts and osteophytes: A Baker cyst describes downwards and backwards herniation of the synovial cavity of the knee, which is usually secondary to osteoarthritis. Surgery (unicompartmental or total joint replacement) is reserved for severe disease that is symptomatic despite regular analgesia.

4. E – Osgood-Schlatter disease

Osgood-Schlatter disease is a condition that is most common in younger teenage boys and is characterized by inflammation of the tibial tubercle. It is caused by a strain on the developing tubercle by the pull of the patellar tendon. Features include pain that is localized to the tubercle and is worse with activity. The pain is particularly prominent on straight leg raise against resistance. On examination, the tibial tubercle may be prominent. Osgood-Schlatter disease is usually self-limiting, so treatment is not required.

Pellegrini-Stieda disease is characterized by ossification of a subligamentous haematoma that occurs after partial avulsion of the medial collateral ligament from the medial condyle of the femur. There is localized thickening and tenderness over the site of ossification.

Robert Bayley Osgood, American orthopaedic surgeon (1873–1956).

Carl Schlatter, Swiss physician (1864–1934).

5. J – Prepatellar bursitis

The prepatellar bursa lies in front of the lower half of the patella and the upper part of the patellar tendon. Repeated friction of the bursa, usually in those who kneel, results in pain and swelling of the bursa. This is known as prepatellar bursitis, or housemaid's knee. Management can be either by aspiration (although recurrence may occur) or by excision of the offending bursa. Vicar's knee has a similar presentation but affects the infrapatellar bursa instead.

THEME 15: DIAGNOSIS OF VASCULAR DISEASE

1. A – Buerger disease

This young man presents with claudication despite having few risk factors for atherosclerosis. In fact, he has Buerger disease, a vasculitis of medium-sized vessels that results in progressive obliteration of distal arteries in young men (<45 years) who smoke heavily. It is most common in Asians and Ashkenazi Jews, and is associated with HLA-B5. Buerger disease affects the upper and lower limbs. The main symptom is pain, but chronic inflammation and thrombosis can result in ulcerations and gangrene, often requiring amputations. Arteriography shows normal proximal vessels and distal occlusions with multiple 'corkscrew' collaterals. Management is with analgesia and stopping smoking. If tobacco use is not ceased, multiple amputations will be unavoidable.

Takayasu arteritis (also known as pulseless disease) is a rare vasculitis characterized by granulomatous inflammation of the aorta and its major branches. Features include hypertension, arm claudication, absent pulses, bruits and visual disturbance (transient ambylopia and blindness). Patients also present with systemic illness (malaise, fever, night sweats and weight loss). It is most common in younger Asian women. Diagnosis is by angiography, which shows narrowing of the aorta and its major branches. Management is with steroids, but the condition is progressive and death occurs within a few years.

Leo Buerger, Austrian-born American physician and urologist (1879–1943).

Mikito Takayasu, Japanese ophthalmologist (1860–1938).

2. D – Embolus

The irregularly irregular heart beat in this woman who presents with an acute cold, pulseless limb suggests embolus-induced acute limb ischaemia from atrial fibrillation. Acute limb ischaemia is a surgical emergency presenting with 'the 6 P's': a pale, painful, paraesthetic, paralyzed, pulseless, perishingly cold limb. Causes include embolism, acute thrombosis, trauma, aortic dissection and intra-arterial injection (iatrogenic or by intravenous drug users).

3. F – Ruptured Baker cyst

This woman has a history of bilateral lower limb osteoarthritis and presents with sudden pain in a calf. The main differentials are a deep vein thrombosis (DVT) or a ruptured Baker cyst secondary to osteoarthritis. With her history and the negative Doppler study, the ruptured cyst is more likely.

A Baker cyst (or popliteal cyst) is a benign swelling that arises between the medial head of the gastrocnemius and the semimembranous muscles behind the knee. Underlying osteoarthritis can cause the synovium of the knee to bulge posteriorly into the popliteal space, where it may be palpable. When the Baker cyst ruptures, it results in acute calf pain and swelling. The diagnosis is confirmed by ultrasound.

William Morrant Baker, English surgeon (1839–1896).

4. I – Superficial thrombophlebitis

Thrombophlebitis is inflammation of a vein following the formation of a thrombus within it. Risk factors for thrombophlebitis include varicose veins, cannula insertion, polycythaemia and Buerger disease. Patients present with pain and erythema with a cord-like inflamed area. Management is by rest, compression and elevation of the limb, along with anti-inflammatory drugs.

5. H – Subclavian steal syndrome

This woman has a cervical rib that is impinging on her right subclavian artery. When the arm is exerted, it requires more blood, but because the subclavian artery is narrowed, the blood has to come from elsewhere, so it is 'stolen' from the vertebral artery, which is meant to supply the brain. This is why, in cases of subclavian artery impingement when the arm is over-used and blood is diverted away from the vertebral artery, a transient loss of consciousness occurs. This is known as the subclavian steal syndrome.

THEME 16: INVESTIGATION OF DYSPHAGIA

1. H – Manometry

Achalasia is a progressive failure of relaxation of the lower oesophagus with dilatation, tortuosity and hypertrophy of the oesophagus above. It occurs secondary to idiopathic degeneration of the nerve ganglia of the oesophagus, known as Auerbach myenteric plexus. Achalasia is most common in the third through fifth decades and is more prevalent in females. Patients experience worsening dysphagia, and regurgitation from the dilated oesophagus can result in aspiration pneumonia. Chest X-ray appearances include the lack of a gastric bubble (because the dilated oesophagus does not empty, so swallowed air cannot pass to the stomach). The dilated oesophageal sac with food in it gives rise to the air–fluid level and the 'double right heart border' appearance.

A barium swallow in achalasia shows a dilated oesophagus with a tapering lower segment resembling a bird's beak. The diagnosis of achalasia is by manometry whereby a catheter containing pressure sensors is passed via the nose into the lower oesophagus and patients are asked to perform a series of swallows. Patients with achalasia exhibit an increased lower oesophageal pressure at rest, failure of the oesophagus to relax after swallowing and the absence of useful peristalsis in the lower oesophagus. Management is by balloon dilatation of the oesophagus or by Heller cardiomyotomy, where the muscle of the oesophagus is cut longitudinally down to the mucosa. Achalasia predisposes to squamous cell carcinoma of the oesophagus.

Ernest Heller, German surgeon (performed first cardiomyotomy in 1913).

2. A – 24-hour lower oesophageal pH

Gastro-oesophageal reflux disease (GORD) results from a low resting tone of the lower oesophageal sphincter and may be associated with a hiatus hernia. Because of this, the oesophageal mucosa is exposed to gastric acid for prolonged periods, resulting in inflammation, ulceration and stricture formation. Risk factors for the development of GORD include obesity, chronic cough, diet (fat, alcohol, coffee) and repeated vomiting. Patients present with heartburn and regurgitation provoked by bending, straining and lying down.

The diagnosis of reflux can be made by measuring the lower oesophageal pH. A pH probe is inserted into the lower oesophagus through the nose and left for 24 hours – if the pH <4 for more than 4 hours then oesophageal reflux is confirmed. Management of reflux can be conservative (weight loss, diet changes and antacids), medical or surgical. Drugs used to manage GORD include proton pump inhibitors (PPIs), such as omeprazole and pantoprazole. Surgical repair of medically resistant reflux is with Nissen fundoplication, where the fundus of the stomach is wrapped around the lower oesophagus.

Rudolph Nissen, German surgeon (1896–1981).

3. K – Tensilon test

Fatigability (movements that gradually get weaker) that is worse at the end of the day is the cardinal feature of myasthenia gravis. Myasthenia gravis is a progressive inability to sustain a maintained or repeated contraction of striated muscle. Affected patients are most often middle-aged females who present with diplopia, ptosis and dysphagia. Myasthenia gravis is caused by autoantibodies to acetylcholine receptors at the postsynaptic neuromuscular junction, thus hindering satisfactory neurotransmission. The diagnosis of myasthenia gravis is made by the Tensilon test, where an intravenous injection of edrophonium bromide (a short-acting anticholinesterase) is shown to transiently improve muscle weakness. Treatment is with anticholinesterases, which inhibit the breakdown of acetylcholine and increase its concentration at the neuromuscular junction. It is a potentially fatal condition if the weakness becomes so severe it affects respiratory muscle function.

4. C – Anti-centromere antibody

Scleroderma can be characterized by the CREST syndrome: Calcinosis, Raynaud, oEsophageal dysmotility, Sclerodactyly and Telangiectasia. This woman has two of the above features, oesophageal dysmotility (manifest as dysphagia) and sclerodactyly (tight skin over the fingers). Systemic features of scleroderma include renal impairment and pulmonary fibrosis. The anti-centromere antibody may be found in patients with the CREST syndrome.

5. J – Serial X-rays

Swallowed foreign bodies can present either with a history of the event or with painful dysphagia. A diagnosis can be confirmed by barium swallow or by X-ray. If a foreign body is lodged in the oesophagus, it can be removed under endoscopy. Foreign bodies that have already passed through the cardia are managed conservatively, with serial X-rays taken to ensure that the foreign body is moving though the gastrointestinal tract. Only foreign bodies that have potential to perforate the bowel need be extracted surgically. This includes batteries (they can break down and release acid) and sharp objects.

THEME 17: UPPER LIMB NERVE LESIONS

The somatic nerve supply to the upper limb is derived from the brachial plexus. This is a quilt work of nerves that is derived from the anterior (ventral) rami of nerve roots C5-T1 (the dorsal rami consist of afferent sensory fibres). The plexus itself can be split into roots, trunks (upper, middle and lower), divisions (anterior and posterior) and cords (posterior, lateral and medial) before delivering its five terminal branches, the musculocutaneous, axillary, median, ulnar and radial nerves.

1. C – Distal median nerve

Compression of the distal portion of the median nerve can occur in the carpal tunnel as it passes behind the flexor retinaculum. Carpal tunnel syndrome is more common in women, during pregnancy and with certain medical conditions such as rheumatoid arthritis, acromegaly and hypothyroidism. Patients experience tingling and numbness in the radial three-and-a-half digits, which may be followed by wasting of the thenar eminence (supplied by the median nerve). Clinical tests that help confirm carpal tunnel syndrome include Tinel test (tapping over the median nerve at the wrist reproduces symptoms) and Phalen test (symptoms are reproduced by holding the wrist palmarflexed for 1 minute).

Proximal lesions of the median nerve (i.e. entrapment before the nerve enters the carpal tunnel) manifest as pain in the anterior aspect of the distal upper arm and forearm with loss of sensation in the radial three-and-a-half digits. Tinel and Phalen tests are negative. Proximal median nerve lesions can occur with forearm fractures and elbow dislocation.

Jules Tinel, French neurologist (1879–1952).

George Phalen, American orthopaedic surgeon (1911–1998).

2. I – Upper brachial plexus

Upper brachial plexus injuries, also known as Erb's palsy, involve the C5 and C6 nerve roots (the brachial plexus is made of the roots C5 to T1). They are commonly caused by traction injuries, such as motorcycle accidents or birth injuries (due to pulling on the baby's arm). There is flaccid paralysis of the arm abductors, lateral rotators of the shoulder and supinators, so the affected arm hangs limp and is medially rotated, extended at the elbow and pronated with the hand pointing backwards – the waiter's tip position. Paralysis is accompanied by loss of sensation over the lateral arm and forearm.

Wilhelm Heinrich Erb, German neurologist (1840–1921).

3. H – Radial nerve

The radial nerve runs in close proximity to the shaft of the humerus in the spiral groove. Common causes of radial nerve palsies include humeral shaft fractures (as in this scenario, in which case patients also suffer bruising to the upper arm), compression of the nerve in the arm with prolonged use of ill-fitting crutches, and elbow dislocations or Monteggia fractures. Damage of the radial nerve is also seen in people who fall asleep with their arm hanging over the back of a chair (Saturday night palsy).

The radial nerve supplies the extensors to the forearm and wrist, and a radial nerve palsy results in an inability to extend the wrist or metacarpophalangeal joints (wrist drop), forearm extensor wasting and a loss of sensation in the anatomical snuffbox. The anatomical snuffbox is the name given to the triangular region on the radial dorsal aspect of the hand at the level of the carpal bones. It is so-called as this was the surface used in the sixteenth century for placing and snorting snuff (powdered tobacco).

4. E – Posterior interosseous nerve

The posterior interosseous nerve is a branch of the radial nerve that runs deep in the forearm to supply the wrist and finger extensors except the extensor carpi radialis longus (which is innervated by a proximal branch from the radial nerve). The posterior interosseous nerve can be damaged in forearm fractures, resulting in an inability to extend the fingers and in a weak wrist drop. The wrist drop is only slight, as the extensor carpi radialis longus muscle still provides some wrist extension. There is no sensory loss with these nerve lesions.

The anterior interosseous nerve is a motor branch of the median nerve in the forearm. Lesions of this nerve are rare, usually arising from deep lacerations to the forearm. The anterior interosseous nerve provides motor fibres to the flexor pollicis longus, the medial part of the flexor digitorum profundus and pronator quadratus. Patients have a weakness in the thumb and index finger characterized by a deformity in the pinch mechanism between the thumb and index finger.

5. D – Distal ulnar nerve

The ulnar nerve is most commonly damaged behind the elbow (proximal lesions) and at the wrist (distal lesions). The ulnar nerve supplies the small muscles of the hand (except the LOAF muscles: Lateral two lumbrical, Opponens pollicis, Abductor pollicis and Flexor pollicis brevis). It also provides sensation to the medial skin of the palm and the back of the hand and to the medial one-and-a-half digits. Ulnar lesions at the wrist result in sensory loss to the ulnar one-and-a-half digits but not to the hand. This is because the branches of the ulnar nerve that supply the skin of the medial hand (i.e. the palmar cutaneous and dorsal cutaneous branches) originate proximal to the wrist. The digital sensory branch originates in the wrist. Ulnar nerve lesions also result in hand weakness. Chronic lesions of the ulnar nerve result in clawing of the hand.

Froment test is used to determine the presence of ulnar nerve lesions. A piece of paper is placed between the thumb and index finger on the affected side and the patient is told to grip the paper. The examiner then tries to remove the paper from between the patient's fingers. Normally, the patient will be able to prevent the paper from being removed by using the adductor pollicis muscle to hold the thumb strongly against the index finger. In ulnar nerve lesions, the adductor pollicis muscle does not work, so the patient instead has to flex the interphalangeal joint of the thumb in order to keep the paper in place. This is a positive Froment test.

Jules Froment, French physician (1878–1946).

Practice Paper 6: Questions

THEME 1: DIAGNOSIS OF HERNIAS

Options

A. Direct inguinal
B. Epigastric
C. Femoral
D. Gastroschisis
E. Hiatus
F. Incisional
G. Indirect inguinal
H. Littré
I. Paraumbilical
J. Spigelian

For each of the following scenarios, select the most likely hernia. Each option may be used once, more than once or not at all.

1. A 57-year-old woman presents to the emergency department with a tender, erythematous swelling in the left groin. On examination, you find an irreducible, hard lump below and lateral to the pubic tubercle.
2. A 24-year-old man presents with a groin swelling that descends into the scrotum on standing. On examination, the swelling does not transilluminate and you cannot get above it, but it is reducible.
3. A 48-year-old woman presents with a 6-month history of heartburn and night cough. She denies any other symptoms. On examination, you note that she is obese, but no other abnormality is evident.
4. A 64-year-old man, who has a history of a laparotomy following a perforated peptic ulcer, presents with a tender mass underlying the caudal end of his midline scar. At operation, the hernial sac is found to contain a Meckel diverticulum.
5. A 52-year-old man presents with a lump in his abdomen that is associated with a dull ache. On examination, the lump is 2 cm in size and below the umbilicus. It is located lateral to the rectus muscles.

THEME 2: SPINAL CORD LESIONS

Options

A. Anterior cord syndrome
B. Brown-Séquard syndrome

C. Cauda equina syndrome
D. Central cord syndrome
E. Posterior cord syndrome
F. Syringomyelia

For each of the following scenarios, select the most likely spinal cord lesion. Each option may be used once, more than once or not at all.

1. A 68-year-old woman attends the emergency department after falling down the stairs. She had suffered trauma to her forehead. On examination, she has bilateral upper limb weakness.
2. A 28-year-old builder falls from scaffolding and hits his head. He describes a hyperextension injury. On examination, there is no motor or sensory dysfunction of the limbs, but the patient evidently has difficulty coordinating his gait.
3. A 19-year-old man is stabbed in the back. He is now unable to move his right lower limb. On examination, you note that he is insensate to pain on the left leg, although motor function in this limb is preserved.
4. A 57-year-old man describes sudden-onset back pain that occurred when trying to lift his sofa earlier in the day. He now complains of an inability to pass urine and of pain going from his back to both his legs. On examination, you note that there is a loss of sensation around the perineum.
5. A 35-year-old woman presents with a long history of worsening neck and shoulder pain associated with sensory loss in both upper limbs. On examination, you note that the patient is insensate to pain and temperature in the distal upper limbs, although joint position sense is intact. There is no other motor or sensory loss.

THEME 3: MANAGEMENT OF BILIARY TRACT DISEASE

Options

A. Antibiotics and elective laparoscopic cholecystectomy
B. Endoscopic retrograde cholangiopancreatogram
C. Laparotomy and cholecystotomy/drainage
D. Magnetic resonance cholangiopancreatogram
E. Medical dissolution therapy
F. Percutaneous gallbladder drainage
G. Ultrasound scan of abdomen

For each of the following presentations, select the most appropriate management. Each option may be used once, more than once or not at all.

1. A 47-year-old woman is seen is the emergency department with a 5-day history of upper abdominal pain, nausea and worsening jaundice. She has experienced bouts of similar pains before, but has never previously had jaundice. On examination, she is apyrexial and there is mild tenderness in the right upper quadrant, but no masses are palpable. An

abdominal ultrasound confirms the presence of a large gallstone in the common bile duct.

2. A 43-year-old woman complains of her first episode of severe epigastric pain, which occurred 2 hours after eating fish and chips. On further questioning, she admits feeling nauseated. There are no other symptoms. Her observations include pulse 96, blood pressure 126/80 and temperature 37°C.
3. A 38-year-old woman presents with a 3-day history of worsening epigastric discomfort. On examination, the abdomen is soft, but she is tender in the epigastrium and right upper quadrant. Her pulse is 96, blood pressure 130/85 and temperature 38.5°C.
4. A 65-year-old woman with known gallstones presents with a 3-day history of severe right upper quadrant pain with nausea and vomiting. On examination, her temperature is 39.1°C. There is tenderness and a palpable mass in the right upper quadrant. A full blood count shows a haemoglobin 11.8 g/dL and leukocytes 27 × 109/L.
5. A 49-year-old woman presents with a 24-hour history of right upper quadrant pain, nausea and vomiting. On examination, she is jaundiced and her temperature is 38.5°C. An abdominal ultrasound shows multiple stones in the gallbladder and a common bile duct diameter of 9 mm.

THEME 4: ULCERS

Options

A. Arterial ulcer
B. Curling ulcer
C. Cushing ulcer
D. Marjolin ulcer
E. Necrobiosis lipoidica
F. Pyoderma gangrenosum
G. Rodent ulcer
H. Syphilitic ulcer
I. Venous ulcer

For each of the following presentations, select the most likely diagnosis. Each option may be used once, more than once or not at all.

1. An 18-year-old man was cycling home without a helmet when he was knocked over by a car. He suffered a severe blow to his head. On admission to the emergency department, the patient had a massive haematemesis and was booked for an urgent endoscopy.
2. A 27-year-old woman presents with a history of diarrhoea associated with the passage of blood and mucus. She claims to feel unwell and tired and to have lost weight in recent months. On examination, you notice a deep, necrotic ulcer on her leg with dark red edges.

3. A 45-year-old man is brought to the emergency department after suffering severe burns in a fire at his home. Five days after his admission to the ward, he complains of passing fresh blood per rectum.
4. A 62-year-old woman presents to her general practitioner with an ulcer on her left ankle. On examination, there is a brownish discolouration of the skin of both ankles and an ulcer over the left medial malleolus.
5. A 30-year-old man attends his general practice diabetic clinic for a routine check-up. He shows the nurse practitioner a lesion on his left shin that has appeared since his previous appointment. On examination, a 3 cm atrophic, yellowish, shiny lesion is identified.

THEME 5: CONSENT

Options

A. Apply to make the child a ward of court
B. Doctor can consent for the patient
C. Doctor can treat patient under duty of care
D. Doctor can treat patient under the Mental Health Act
E. Daughter's refusal to treatment is valid
F. Parents' refusal to treatment is valid
G. Patient can give valid consent to treatment
H. Patient's refusal is invalid and can be overridden
I. Patient's refusal is valid and cannot be overridden

For each of the following presentations, select the most appropriate course of action. Each option may be used once, more than once or not at all.

1. A 26-year-old man is admitted to hospital with testicular torsion. He has a past medical history of severe depression for which he is under Section. The patient refuses surgery, even though he understands the benefits of having surgery and the risks of not going to theatre.
2. A 72-year-old man is admitted after a fall. He is found to have a fracture of his left femur, for which he needs operative treatment. The patient has severe dementia, with an Abbreviated Mental Test Score of 2. His daughter is refusing treatment on his behalf.
3. A 13-year-old boy is admitted with right iliac fossa pain and vomiting. He is thought to have appendicitis and is scheduled for surgery. The boy understands the complications and benefits of removing his appendix and the risks of non-operative intervention. Despite this, he is refusing operative intervention although his parents are adamant that he should go to theatre.
4. A 72-year-old man with known metastatic thyroid cancer is admitted to hospital with worsening shortness of breath and a cough. By the time of his admission to the ward, he is unconscious, and it is suggested that artificial ventilation is required. His daughter shows you an advance directive that the patient had made expressing a wish not to have any medical intervention should he become critically ill.

5. A 15-year-old boy with severe learning difficulties is brought to the emergency department with worsening shortness of breath. A routine blood test shows profound anaemia requiring blood transfusion. His parents are refusing to the proposed management, saying that it is up to God to decide whether or not their child gets better.

THEME 6: COLORECTAL OPERATIONS

Options

A. Abdominoperineal resection
B. Anterior resection
C. Extended right hemicolectomy
D. Hartmann procedure
E. Left hemicolectomy
F. Proctocolectomy and ileo-anal pouch
G. Right hemicolectomy
H. Sigmoid colectomy
I. Stricturoplasty

For each of the following scenarios, select the most appropriate operation. Each option may be used once, more than once or not at all.

1. A 62-year-old woman with known diverticular disease of the sigmoid colon presents with sudden-onset abdominal pain and vomiting. On examination, the abdomen is rigid. An erect chest X-ray confirms air under the diaphragm.
2. A 64-year-old man presents with rectal bleeding and a feeling of incomplete emptying after defaecation. A per rectum examination reveals a tumour 1 cm from the anal margin.
3. A 65-year-old woman who presented with rectal bleeding is found to have a non-obstructing tumour of the sigmoid colon.
4. A 74-year-old woman presents with weight loss and rectal bleeding. An urgent colonoscopy reveals a non-obstructive tumour at the caecum.
5. A 70-year-old woman who was found to have anaemia on her last admission to hospital has a lower gastrointestinal endoscopy arranged. She is found to have a high rectal tumour.

THEME 7: MANAGEMENT OF BREAST CANCER

Options

A. Adjuvant chemotherapy
B. Aromatase inhibitor
C. Modified radical mastectomy
D. Neoadjuvant chemotherapy
E. Radiotherapy
F. Tamoxifen
G. Trastuzumab

H. Wide local excision and axillary clearance
I. Wide local excision and sentinel node biopsy

For each of the following people presenting with breast cancer, select the most appropriate management plan. Each option may be used once, more than once or not at all.

1. A 32-year-old woman is found to have a 5 cm invasive ductal carcinoma in the upper outer quadrant. You have explained that she may need a mastectomy, but she is keen to preserve the breast.
2. A 65-year-old woman has a 6.5 cm central invasive breast tumour. She is otherwise fit and well.
3. A 42-year-old woman has recently had a wide local excision and axillary clearance for a 2 cm breast carcinoma. Histology showed clear excision margins, a grade I oestrogen receptor-negative tumour and no positive axillary lymph nodes. She returns to the outpatient clinic and wants to know what further treatment she will be having.
4. A 35-year-old woman who has recently had a 3 cm invasive breast tumour resection has returned to clinic. The histology report states that the tumour is oestrogen receptor-negative but is overexpressing HER2.
5. A 64-year-old woman has just had a radical mastectomy and radiotherapy for a large invasive breast tumour. Histology showed an oestrogen receptor-positive tumour. Apart from suffering a left deep vein thrombosis during the postoperative recovery period, she is well.

THEME 8: TUMOUR STAGING SYSTEMS

Options

A. Ann Arbor
B. Breslow
C. Dukes A
D. Dukes B
E. Dukes C
F. Dukes D
G. Gleason

For each of the following scenarios, choose the most appropriate tumour staging/staging system. Each option may be used once, more than once or not at all.

1. A 67-year-old man presents with difficulty passing urine. He has an elevated prostate-specific antigen, and a transrectal biopsy is performed.
2. A 72-year-old man has a sigmoid tumour resected. The pathologist notes that the tumour is confined to the bowel wall and that there is no lymph node involvement.

3. A 45-year-old man presents with a 4-week history of fever, night sweats and itching. He has lost 5 kg in weight over the last fortnight. On examination, enlarged lymph nodes are palpable in the neck.
4. A 65-year-old woman has a colon tumour resected successfully. The pathology report states that the tumour has invaded the bowel wall. The preoperative CT scan shows multiple metastases in the liver.
5. A 27-year-old woman presents with an irregularly pigmented lesion on her lower right leg that is subsequently excised.

THEME 9: INVESTIGATION OF ENDOCRINE DISEASE

Options

A. 17-Hydroxyprogesterone levels
B. 24-hour urinary vanillylmandelic acid
C. 24-hour urinary 5-hydroxyindole acetic acid
D. Aldosterone and renin levels
E. Dexamethasone suppression test
F. Parathyroid hormone and calcium levels
G. Serum calcitonin
H. Short Synacthen test
I. Vitamin D levels

For each of the following people, select the best distinguishing investigation. Each option may be used once, more than once or not at all.

1. A 42-year-old man is referred to the general medical clinic by his general practitioner for uncontrollable hypertension. He is presently on ramipril and bendroflumethiazide. On further questioning, he admits to having paroxysms of anxiety, sweating and palpitations that are brought on by stress, which he describes as 'panic attacks'.
2. A 44-year-old woman presents following a faint after standing up from a sitting position. She did not lose consciousness during this episode, but reported feeling 'dizzy and lightheaded'. She has no significant past medical history. On examination, you notice multiple areas of skin depigmentation but increased pigmentation in the palmar creases and on the elbows.
3. A 65-year-old woman with known small cell lung cancer presents with hirsutism that she finds embarrassing. On examination, you note that she has a plethoric face, acne, abdominal striae and multiple bruises.
4. A 5-year-old girl is referred to the paediatric clinic by her general practitioner with precocious puberty. On examination, she is found to have clitoromegaly and some pubic hair. She is above the 98th centile for height and weight.
5. A 50-year-old man attends the emergency department complaining of episodes of flushing and diarrhoea associated with difficulty breathing.

On further questioning, you find that these episodes are precipitated by stress and alcohol. On examination, his blood pressure is 130/86 mmHg and heart rate 82/min.

THEME 10: DIAGNOSIS OF DYSPHAGIA

Options

A. Achalasia
B. Boerhaave syndrome
C. Diffuse oesophageal spasm
D. External oesophageal compression
E. Foreign body
F. Hiatus hernia
G. Mallory-Weiss tear
H. Myasthenia gravis
I. Oesophageal carcinoma
J. Oesophageal web
K. Pharyngeal pouch

For each of the following people presenting with dysphagia, select the most likely diagnosis. Each option may be used once, more than once or not at all.

1. A 46-year-old woman presents to the general practitioner with worsening dysphagia for solids. On examination, you notice that her tongue is smooth and she has deformed nails. Routine blood tests show a haemoglobin level of 9.0 g/dL (normal range 11.5–16.0 g/dL), with a mean cell volume of 70 fL (normal range 76–96 fL).
2. A 67-year-old man presents with dysphagia and a night cough – symptoms he has suffered for 6 months. He has recently been admitted to hospital with a chest infection. On examination, there is a soft swelling in the anterior triangle of the neck that gurgles on palpation.
3. A 72-year-old woman presents with dysphagia and worsening shortness of breath. On examination, her pulse is irregularly irregular. She has a flushed face, and auscultation reveals a mid-diastolic murmur.
4. A 57-year-old woman presents with occasional retrosternal pain and acid reflux. She denies other symptoms and examination is unremarkable. A chest X-ray shows an air–fluid level behind the heart.
5. A 48-year-old man presents with sudden-onset pain in his chest and neck with dysphagia. On examination, he appears unwell. An ECG shows no acute changes and cardiac enzymes are normal. A chest X-ray shows gas in the mediastinum.

THEME 11: MANAGEMENT OF URINARY RETENTION

Options

A. Check urea and electrolytes

B. Cystoscopy
C. Intravenous antibiotics
D. Lithotripsy
E. Percutaneous nephrostomy
F. Reassurance alone
G. Suprapubic catheterization
H. Transurethral resection of prostate
I. Trial without catheter
J. Urethral catheterization

For each of the following patients presenting with urinary retention, select the most appropriate management. Each option may be used once, more than once or not at all.

1. A 64-year-old man presents with suprapubic pain and a sudden inability to pass urine. On examination, there is a palpable suprapubic mass that is dull to percussion. A bladder scan demonstrates 750 mL in the bladder.
2. A 64-year-old man presents with suprapubic pain and a sudden inability to pass urine. On examination, there is a palpable suprapubic mass that is dull to percussion. This was preceded by a 4-week history of passage of frank haematuria, including the occasional clot. Three failed attempts have been made at urethral catheterization.
3. A 64-year-old man presents with suprapubic pain and a sudden inability to pass urine. On examination, there is a palpable suprapubic mass that is dull to percussion. There is no significant past medical or surgical history. Three failed attempts have been made at urethral catheterization.
4. A 64-year-old man presents with suprapubic pain and a sudden inability to pass urine. On examination, there is a palpable suprapubic mass that is dull to percussion. A urethral catheter is passed successfully and a 500 mL residual volume is recorded. You see the patient the next day on the ward round, and he asks you what will happen next.
5. A 64-year-old man presents with a history of overflow incontinence. He does not complain of any pain and is still able to empty his bladder, although this takes some time and there is dribbling at the end of the stream. On examination, the bladder is palpable 5 fingerbreaths above the pubis.

THEME 12: DIAGNOSIS OF PAEDIATRIC SURGICAL CONDITIONS

Options

A. Appendicitis
B. Duodenal atresia
C. Exomphalos
D. Gastroschisis
E. Hirschprung disease
F. Intussusception
G. Meckel diverticulum

H. Mesenteric adenitis
I. Necrotizing enterocolitis
J. Pyloric stenosis

For each of the following presentations, select the most likely diagnosis. Each option may be used once, more than once or not at all.

1. A newborn baby presents with bile-stained vomiting and abdominal distension on its third day of life. An abdominal X-ray reveals gas in the stomach and the first part of the duodenum, but nowhere else in the abdomen.
2. A 2-day-old baby presents with abdominal distension and bile-stained vomiting. It is noted that she has failed to pass meconium. An abdominal X-ray shows enlarged small and large bowel loops.
3. A baby is born with its liver and some small intestine herniating through a defect in the anterior abdominal wall adjacent to the umbilicus.
4. A 9-year-old boy presents with a 2-day history of right iliac fossa pain, nausea and vomiting, anorexia, and diarrhoea. On examination, the boy is tender in the right iliac fossa, with no masses palpable. His temperature is 37.8°C.
5. A 6-year-old girl presents with an episode of painless rectal bleeding. She complains of no other symptoms and she otherwise feels well. Rectal examination shows no obvious abnormality.

THEME 13: DIAGNOSIS OF FOOT DISORDERS

Options

A. Claw-toe
B. Freiberg disease
C. Gout
D. Hallux rigidus
E. Hallux valgus
F. Hammer toe
G. Mallet toe
H. March fracture
I. Morton's neuralgia
J. Pseudogout
K. Sever disease

For each of the following people presenting with foot problems, select the most likely diagnosis. Each option may be used once, more than once or not at all.

1. A 64-year-old man presents with sudden-onset severe pain in his left toe that occurred at rest. He is otherwise well. On examination, the small joint of the great toe is swollen, red and tender. The patient is unable to move the joint because of the pain.

2. A 38-year-old man presents with a history of pain over the dorsum of the foot. The pain is sharp and located to the cleft between the third and fourth toes on the right side.
3. A 14-year-old boy presents with left heel pain that has been stopping him playing football for 2 weeks. On examination, there is tenderness localized over the calcaneum near the insertion of the Achilles tendon.
4. A 28-year-old woman presents with a recent history of pain in her right foot, especially on walking. She has joined the army, and the pain is preventing her from participating in military activities. On examination, there is a swelling over the second metatarsal.
5. A 52-year-old woman presents with a long history of pain in both of her big toes. On examination, both affected toes are deviated laterally and there is a tender swelling of the metatarsophalangeal joints.

THEME 14: DIAGNOSIS OF ABDOMINAL PAIN

Options

A. Acute appendicitis
B. Acute pancreatitis
C. Acute radiation enterocolitis
D. Chronic radiation enterocolitis
E. Diverticulitis
F. Ectopic pregnancy
G. Irritable bowel syndrome
H. Mesenteric angina
I. Osler-Weber-Rendu syndrome
J. Pelvic inflammatory disease
K. Perforated peptic ulcer
L. Subphrenic abscess
M. Torsion of an ovarian cyst

For each of the following people presenting with abdominal pain, select the most likely diagnosis. Each option may be used once, more than once or not at all.

1. An 18-year-old woman is seen with a 48-hour history of lower abdominal pain, vomiting and diarrhoea. On examination, there is tenderness and guarding in the right iliac fossa and no masses are palpable. A routine urinary β-hCG test is negative.
2. A 54-year-old woman presents with sudden-onset abdominal pain that she describes as moderately severe. She has a history of recurrent nose bleeds. On examination, you notice multiple telangiectasias around her mouth. Abdominal examination is unremarkable.
3. A 74-year-old man attends his general practice with a 3-month history of central, aching abdominal pain. The pain occurs soon after eating and

can last up to half an hour. Because of this, the patient has avoided eating and has lost a stone in weight.

4. A 34-year-old man who is currently undergoing treatment for a testicular tumour presents with a 2-day history of cramping abdominal pain, nausea, anorexia and diarrhoea. He denies any infectious contacts or eating 'dodgy' food. A stool culture comes back as negative.
5. A 32-year-old woman is brought to the emergency department by her husband with a sudden-onset, severe abdominal pain. On examination, there is guarding over the lower abdomen. The patient's pulse is 125, blood pressure 86/56 and temperature 36.5°C.

THEME 15: MANAGEMENT OF HEAD INJURY

Options

A. Admit for neurological observation
B. CT head scan
C. Home with written advice
D. Intubation and ventilation
E. Refer to neurosurgery

For each of the following people presenting with head injury, select the most appropriate management. Each option may be used once, more than once or not at all.

1. A 43-year-old man fell down the stairs at home and hit his head on the bottom step. His son, who witnessed the fall, said that the man lost consciousness for about a minute. The patient does not have amnesia and his Glasgow Coma Score (GCS) is 15.
2. A 32-year-old man is hit on the head with a lamp during a robbery. He feels well apart from pain at the site of injury. A skull X-ray shows a depressed fracture.
3. A 65-year-old woman falls at home. On arrival she appears well, but it is apparent that she has been drinking. She has a large laceration to her head, and a skull X-ray shows a hairline fracture on the left side.
4. A 22-year-old woman is involved in a road traffic accident. On arrival at the emergency department, she is unresponsive and makes no response to painful stimuli. She has a swelling over the left temporal region.
5. A 28-year-old man banged his head during a cycling accident. He was not wearing a helmet. On arrival at hospital, his GCS is 15. The examining doctor notices that the patient has straw-coloured fluid leaking from his nose.

THEME 16: UROLOGICAL CONDITIONS

Options

A. Acute cystitis
B. Anticoagulation therapy

C. Benign prostatic hyperplasia
D. Bladder neck stenosis
E. Nephroblastoma
F. Polycystic kidney disease
G. Prostate carcinoma
H. Pyelonephritis
I. Renal cell carcinoma
J. Renal tract calculi
K. Transitional cell carcinoma of the bladder

For each of the following scenarios, select the most appropriate diagnosis. Each option may be used once, more than once or not at all.

1. A 67-year-old man presents with sudden-onset back pain that occurred while walking. He has been having difficulty passing urine over the past few months and admits to terminal dribbling. On examination, there is dullness to percussion in the suprapubic region.
2. An 18-year-old woman presents with a 24-hour history of burning sensation on micturation. She has also been passing water more frequently than usual. On examination, she is tender suprapubically, but there is no tenderness in either renal angle.
3. A 76-year-old man presents with malaise and a long history of difficulty in voiding urine. Abdominal examination is normal except for a suprapubic mass that is dull to percussion. A per rectum exam reveals a large, smooth prostate gland.
4. A 64-year-old man presents with difficulty voiding and a weak stream. He had similar symptoms 6 years ago, and the underlying cause was found to be benign prostatic hyperplasia, for which he had a transurethral resection of the prostate. Abdominal examination was normal and per rectum examination demonstrated no mass.
5. A 12-month-old boy is brought to the general practice by his mother with irritability, fever and occasional blood in the nappy. On examination, a large mass is felt on the left side of the abdomen. The child has dropped two centile lines for weight and height over the last 6 months.

THEME 17: MANAGEMENT OF ABDOMINAL AORTIC ANEURYSMS

Options

A. CT scan
B. Emergency surgery
C. Elective endoluminal repair
D. Elective open repair
E. Urgent elective repair
F. Ultrasound in 6 months
G. Ultrasound in 1 year

For each of the following scenarios, select the most appropriate management plan. Each option may be used once, more than once or not at all.

1. A 67-year-old man presents with sudden-onset epigastric pain radiating to the back. He is sweating and feels nauseated. On examination, his pulse is 115/min and blood pressure 90/55 mmHg.
2. A 62-year-old man presents with renal colic. On reporting a CT of his renal tract, the radiologist notes the presence of a 3 cm infrarenal aortic aneurysm.
3. A 68-year-old man presents with renal colic. On reporting a CT of his renal tract, the radiologist notes the presence of a 5 cm infrarenal aortic aneurysm.
4. A 72-year-old man attends outpatients for his regular abdominal aortic ultrasound. On this occasion, his aortic diameter is 5.9 cm. This compares with 4.2 cm 6 months previously.
5. A 68-year-old man with a known abdominal aortic aneurysm (AAA) presents for a follow-up ultrasound scan. Over the last year, his aneurysm has grown from 5.2 cm to 6.0 cm. The ultrasound scan demonstrates an AAA extending from 1 cm below the renal arteries.

Practice Paper 6: Answers

THEME 1: DIAGNOSIS OF HERNIAS

1. C – Femoral

The femoral triangle is found on the upper thigh just below the inguinal ligament, and contains, from lateral to medial, the femoral nerve, femoral artery and femoral vein (remember 'NAVY': Nerve, Artery, Vein, Y-fronts). The femoral canal is a space just medial to the femoral vein that contains fat, lymph nodes and vessels. It is into this potential space that femoral hernias can protrude.

Femoral hernias are the third most common spontaneous hernia, occurring most frequently in older, multiparous women (this is because the femoral ring is larger in females and pregnancy stretches the fascia over the femoral canal). Noten howevern that inguinal herniae are still more common than femoral herniae in this subpopulation. They protrude through the narrow femoral ring and into the femoral canal, where they expand considerably. On examination, femoral hernias are below and lateral to the pubic tubercle, and the right side is affected twice as commonly as the left. Because the neck of the femoral ring is narrow, there is a high risk of strangulation (50% at 1 month); thus all femoral hernias should be operated on urgently.

2. G – Indirect inguinal

The inguinal canal is 4 cm long and passes downwards and medially from the deep inguinal ring (an inch above the midpoint of the inguinal ligament) to the superficial inguinal ring (an inch above the pubic tubercle). An indirect hernia is one that travels down the inguinal canal and into the scrotum. They occur lateral to the inferior epigastric vessels.

Indirect inguinal hernias are the most common type of hernia and occur most often in young, active men and premature babies (as the processus vaginalis is more likely to be patent). Indirect inguinal hernias are also more common on the right side, because the right testicle descends later and there is a greater incidence of failed closure of the processus vaginalis. On examination, the hernia lies above and medial to the pubic tubercle, and may be observed to descend into the scrotum on standing or coughing. It does not transilluminate, nor is the examiner able to palpate

the upper border of the lump. The principles of surgical repair include defining the anatomy, identifying and reducing the hernia, and closing the defect (usually in the form of a prosthetic mesh).

3. E – Hiatus

A hiatus hernia describes the protrusion of the upper part of the stomach into the thorax through a defect in the diaphragm. There are three types: (1) a sliding hernia (95% of cases) – where the gastro-oesophageal junction (GOJ) is pulled up into the thorax; (2) a rolling hernia (5%) – where the GOJ remains in place but a portion of the fundus of the stomach herniates adjacent to the GOJ; and (3) a mixed type with elements of both sliding and rolling hernias (rare).

Hiatus hernias are more common in obese, older women and the majority are asymptomatic. Features of hiatus hernias include acid reflux, waterbrash (reflex salivation secondary to acid reflux into the lower oesophagus), a night cough (due to refluxed acid tracking to the proximal oesophagus on lying down) and dysphagia. They are also associated with Barrett oesophagus. A chest X-ray may demonstrate an air–fluid level within the hernia behind the heart, but a gastroscopy would be the best determining investigation. Sliding hernias are managed with symptomatic treatments (e.g. proton pump inhibitors). Rolling hiatus hernias require urgent surgical repair (Nissen fundoplication) due to the risk of a complete gastric volvulus. Laparoscopic repair is now preferred due to an improved recovery time.

4. H – Littré

Littré hernia is one that contains a Meckel diverticulum.

Alexis Littré, French anatomist (1685–1726).

5. J – Spigelian

A Spigelian hernia (or spontaneous lateral ventral hernia) describes herniation through the semilunar line, which is a curved tendinous insertion that corresponds to the lateral border of the rectus abdominis muscle and is formed by the aponeuroses of the internal oblique, external oblique and transverses muscles. They tend to occur below the level of the umbilicus. Spigelian hernias are small and develop in the over-50 population. They can present with diffuse pain around the area. There is a high risk of strangulation, so these hernias should be repaired.

Adriaan van den Spiegel, Flemish anatomist (1578–1625).

THEME 2: SPINAL CORD LESIONS

In general, the spinal cord is made up of three tracts on either side. A useful, simplified model of the spinal cord is as follows: the spinothalamic tract makes up the anterior third of the spinal cord and provides pain and temperature fibres to the contralateral side. The corticospinal tract is the middle third of the spinal cord and provides motor fibres to the ipsilateral side. Finally, the dorsal columns are found along the posterior length of the spinal cord and provide vibration sense and proprioception to the ipsilateral side.

1. D – Central cord syndrome

Central cord syndrome is the most common spinal cord lesion. It occurs in older people with cervical spondylosis who sustain a hyperextension injury. There is a flaccid weakness of the arms, but motor and sensory fibres to the lower limb are comparatively preserved as these are located more peripherally in the spinal cord. Central cord lesions have a fair prognosis. The pathogenesis describes a vascular insufficiency from the anterior spinal artery. The artery supplies the central part of the cord. The arrangement of the motor fibres of the cervical cord causes the upper limbs to be most severely affected.

2. E – Posterior cord syndrome

Hyperextension injuries can result in loss of dorsal column function (posterior cord syndrome). These injuries are very rare and the motor and sensory function is preserved. Gait is impaired due to impaired proprioception. The prognosis of posterior cord lesions is good.

The anterior cord syndrome occurs secondary to a flexion-compression injury. There is loss of neurological function of the anterior two-thirds of the spinal cord, namely the spinothalamic (pain and temperature) and corticospinal (motor) tracts. There is greater motor loss in the legs than the arms. The anterior cord syndrome has the worst prognosis of all spinal cord lesions.

3. B – Brown-Séquard syndrome

Brown-Séquard syndrome describes the features of unilateral transection (hemisection) of the spinal cord. Affected patients suffer ipsilateral loss of motor function with impaired joint position and vibration sense (dorsal column dysfunction). There is also a contralateral sensory loss for pain and temperature. Brown-Séquard syndrome has the best prognosis of all spinal cord lesions.

Charles-Édouard Brown-Séquard, British neurologist (1817–1894).

4. C – Cauda equina syndrome

The spinal cord ends around the level of the junction between L1 and L2. Beyond this lies a bundle-like structure of spinal nerve roots known as the cauda equina. If narrowing of the spinal canal occurs below the level of L2 (e.g. in central cord prolapse or from compression by a tumour), then the spinal nerve roots are compromised and the cauda equina syndrome results. Features of cauda equina syndrome include a triad of bowel/bladder disturbance (retention or incontinence), bilateral leg pain and weakness, and loss of sensation in the saddle area (around the perineum). Cauda equina syndrome is considered an emergency and requires urgent decompression either medically or surgically.

Cauda equina, from Latin *cauda* 'tail' and *equus* 'horse'.

5. F – Syringomyelia

Syringomyelia describes the presence of a longitudinal fluid cavity (syrinx) within the spinal cord. These cavities are usually in the cervical segments and disrupt the spinothalamic tracts. Patients present in their 20s–30s with a segmental dissociated loss of spinothalamic function (i.e. spinothalamic function above and below the lesion is preserved). Dorsal column and motor function remain intact. When a syrinx affects the brainstem, the condition is called syringobulbia. Diagnosis of syringomyelia is by MRI and management is by surgical decompression of the syrinx.

Syringomyelia may be associated with an Arnold-Chiari malformation – congenital herniation of the cerebellar tonsils through the foramen magnum at the base of the skull. Syringomyelia may also be caused by tumours of, or trauma to, the spinal cord.

Syrinx, from Greek *syringos* = tube; the word 'syringe' also derives from this.

Julius Arnold, German pathologist (1835–1915).

Hans Chiari, German pathologist (1851–1916).

THEME 3: MANAGEMENT OF BILIARY TRACT DISEASE

1. B – Endoscopic retrograde cholangiopancreatogram

This woman has features of biliary colic and obstructive jaundice due to a stone in the common bile duct (CBD). Since there is no evidence of infection, the most likely diagnosis is choledocholithiasis. Bile duct stones may be silent or present with features of biliary colic (see below). The obstruction of the common bile duct by the stone can result in pale stools and dark urine, as less bile is able to enter the intestine, and more is excreted in the urine. The features of choledocholithiasis remain until the stone disimpacts or passes into the duodenum. If the obstruction is not relieved, the backpressure of bile results in secondary biliary cirrhosis and liver failure. Although some common bile duct stones pass spontaneously, a large stone will need to be removed by endoscopic retrograde cholangiopancreatography (ERCP). Following this, the patient should have her liver function tests and inflammatory markers rechecked before discharge and be placed on the waiting list for an elective cholecystectomy.

Choledocholithiasis, from Latin *chole* = bile + *doch* = duct + *lith* = stone; 'stone in the bile duct'.

ERCP involves cannulation of the biliary tree using a duodenoscope that has a sideways facing camera. The endoscope is used to visualize the major duodenal papilla which marks the entrance to the ampulla of Vater (the confluence of the ventral pancreatic duct and the common bile duct) and biliary tree. This entrance is guarded by the sphincter of Oddi.

Contrast is subsequently injected through this sphincter and X-rays taken to image the biliary tree and any potential abnormalities.

In addition to from being a diagnostic procedure, ERCP can be therapeutic. For example, a stone in the bile duct can be removed or a stent inserted into an area of stricture (i.e. in malignant biliary tree obstruction). Complications of ERCP include pancreatitis (2%), septicaemia, bile duct perforation and contrast reactions. If there is no intended therapeutic need for an ERCP and only imaging is required then a magnetic resonance cholangiopancreatogram (MRCP) is the initial investigation of choice, as it is non-invasive.

2. G – Ultrasound scan of abdomen

Biliary colic occurs when a stone becomes stuck in the cystic duct or at the outlet of the gallbladder, an area known as Hartmann's pouch. The pain of biliary colic is caused by contractions of the smooth muscle of the gallbladder. These contractions can cause the stones to either fall back into the gallbladder or be forced out into the common bile duct. Biliary colic presents as a sudden, severe right upper quadrant pain that lasts for around 2 hours (hence it is not a typical intestinal colicky pain that lasts for 3–5 minutes). The pain can radiate to the right scapula and is exacerbated by eating fatty foods, because fatty foods release the hormone cholecystokinin, which causes the gallbladder to contract against the obstructing stone. On examination, there is tenderness and guarding in the right upper quadrant, which may be accompanied by sweating and tachycardia. Often the patient is restless and cannot keep still with the pain. Patients with biliary colic may get intermittent jaundice as a stone passes out of the cystic duct and into the common bile duct, resulting in a transient obstruction of bile flow. If biliary colic is suspected, an abdominal ultrasound should be performed to confirm the presence of gallstones. Management is with strong analgesia, such as pethidine. Morphine is avoided as it may cause sphincter of Oddi contraction and exacerbate the symptoms. First-line treatment is with NSAIDs unless contraindicated. An elective cholecystectomy should be performed at 6 weeks.

3. A – Antibiotics and elective laparoscopic cholecystectomy

If a gallstone becomes impacted in the neck of the gallbladder, the stasis of bile within the organ can irritate it, resulting in inflammation. This is acute cholecystitis. Acute cholecystitis presents with right upper quadrant pain that increases gradually in severity and that radiates to the tip of the right shoulder blade. The pain is exacerbated by moving and breathing. Pain may be accompanied by nausea, vomiting, anorexia, fever and a high white cell count. On examination, pressing over the gallbladder (at the right costal margin in the midclavicular line) while the patient is in inspiration will cause a 'catching' pain as the gallbladder pushes against your fingers. This is Murphy's sign, and is only positive if a similar manoeuvre does not induce pain on the left side. When pain radiates to the tip of the right shoulder, an area of skin below the scapula may be hypersensitive. This is known as Boas' sign. Although most cases of acute cholecystitis are due to stones, 5% are 'acalculous', i.e. no gallstones are present. Typhoid infection, sepsis, burns and diabetes are examples of causes of acalculous cholecystitis. Ninety percent of cases of acute cholecystitis are relieved with bed rest, fluids, analgesia and intravenous antibiotics. An elective cholecystectomy is then performed after 6 weeks. If symptoms do not settle with conservative management, an emergency cholecystectomy may be performed.

John Benjamin Murphy, American surgeon (1857–1916).

Ismar Isidor Boas, German physician (1858–1938).

4. F – Percutaneous gallbladder drainage

This patient with known gallstones has a high fever, leukocytosis, abdominal pain and a right upper quadrant mass. She has an empyema of the gallbladder. An empyema is the presence of pus in a pre-existing body cavity (as opposed to an abscess, which is pus within a newly formed capsule). If a stone becomes lodged in the gallbladder outlet with existing infection then an empyema can result and the gallbladder may be palpable. If an empyema of the gallbladder is suspected then urgent drainage of the gallbladder should be performed. Options include a laparotomy with drainage of the gallbladder or percutaneous gallbladder drainage. Of the two, radiologically guided percutaneous drainage is the better option, as it avoids potentially life-threatening surgery.

5. B – Endoscopic retrograde cholangiopancreatogram

This woman is presenting with features of Charcot's triad of ascending cholangitis, namely jaundice, fever and right upper quadrant pain. Since she has a dilated common bile duct (normal diameter 6–7 mm), it is likely that an obstructing stone in the distal CBD has caused the disease process. Management would require drainage of the pus in the biliary tree by performing a therapeutic ERCP and removing the offending stone.

THEME 4: ULCERS

1. C – Cushing ulcer

Cushing ulcer (also known as Rokitansky-Cushing syndrome) is the association of peptic ulceration and/or haemorrhage with intracranial injury or raised intracranial pressure. They are typically deep solitary ulcers that are prone to perforation.

Harvey Cushing, American neurosurgeon (1869–1939).

Karl von Rokitansky, Austrian pathologist (1804–1878).

2. F – Pyoderma gangrenosum

Pyoderma gangrenosum is a skin condition with an underlying vasculitis that is associated with inflammatory bowel disease (as in this patient), rheumatoid arthritis and myeloid blood dyscrasias (e.g. acute and chronic myeloid leukaemias). It initially appears as purple papules that enlarge and break down to become deep, necrotic ulcers with a dark red hypertrophic border. Pyoderma gangrenosum is most common on the legs, but can develop anywhere.

3. B – Curling ulcer

Curling ulcer is an acute ulcer of the duodenum that occurs a few days following severe burns. It occurs because the reduced plasma volume results in necrosis of the gastric mucosa, with ensuing ulceration and perforation.

Thomas Blizard Curling, British surgeon (1811–1888).

4. I – Venous ulcer

Venous ulcers occur most often in women after middle age. They occur against a background of deep venous insufficiency. There are many stages of skin changes in venous disease, beginning with oedema and a brown discolouration of the skin. The brown colour comes from haemosiderin deposits that occur secondary to extravasation of red cells from leaky capillaries. The next stages are an eczema-like appearance, with hardening and constriction of the skin around the ankle (lipodermatosclerosis). The tightening of the skin around the ankle that occurs with lipodermatosclerosis, along with the oedema of the leg proximal to this, results in an 'inverted champagne bottle' appearance.

Ulceration of the affected skin often follows trauma and usually affects the medial gaiter area (the gaiter area stretches from the ankle to the proximal calf, much like the gaiters used when hiking to stop boots getting muddy water in them). Treatment involves the application of compression bandages and encouraging movement.

5. E – Necrobiosis lipoidica

Also known as necrobiosis lipoidica diabeticorum, this condition begins as small, raised, red areas that gradually grow to become large, flat, waxy lesions that are reddish-brown or yellow in colour. Necrobiosis lipoidica usually occurs on the shins. The condition is characterized by necrosis of the connective tissue with infiltration of lymphocytes and granulocytes. Degenerating collagen fibres are replaced with lipid material. Although most patients who develop necrobiosis lipoidica are diabetic, only 1% of diabetics have this condition.

THEME 5: CONSENT

1. I – Patient's refusal is valid and cannot be overridden

This patient understands the risks and benefits of surgery and as such, can be deemed to have capacity to make an informed decision, irrespective of his chronic mental health problems. The Mental Health Act does not allow for treatment of any medical condition other than a psychiatric disorder. His refusal of treatment is therefore valid and the doctor cannot override it.

2. C – Doctor can treat patient under duty of care

This man with dementia requires operative intervention but does not have the capacity to consent. Although his daughter does not wish for him to have the operation, one adult cannot consent for another, whether a relative or a medical professional. In such cases, it is up to the doctor to initiate treatment according to the patient's best interests under the duty of care law.

3. H – Patient's refusal is invalid and can be overridden

This child has capacity to make an informed choice and is thus 'Gillick competent'. A child under 16 years is Gillick competent if he/she understands the implications and complications of a treatment option, whatever their age. A Gillick competent child can consent to treatment without permission from a parent or guardian. However, they cannot refuse treatment. In this case, although the child refuses treatment, operative management can still proceed.

4. I – Patient's refusal is valid and cannot be overridden

This patient is unconscious and cannot currently consent to treatment. If this was the only information the doctor had, he would be able to treat the patient under duty of care. However, if a signed, witnessed advance directive has been made while the patient was competent then the wishes of the patient not to have medical treatment should be respected.

5. A – Apply to make the child a ward of court

This child has learning difficulties and would not qualify as Gillick competent. His parents are refusing treatment on religious grounds although the doctors have suggested that transfusion is necessary. In this case, either the doctor can respect the parents' wishes or can apply to make the child a ward of the High Court. The Court could then override the parents' refusal to treatment.

THEME 6: COLORECTAL OPERATIONS

1. D – Hartmann's procedure

This woman has developed peritonitis following perforation of a diverticulum. She will require an appropriate resection (a sigmoid colectomy) with a delayed anastomosis, known as Hartmann procedure. This procedure involves forming a colostomy and oversewing the rectum which is left inside. This operation avoids the potential complications of forming an anastomosis under suboptimal emergency conditions, and the colostomy can be reversed at a later date, although this is not always performed. Hartmann procedures are usually performed for either perforating diverticulitis or for palliation of colorectal cancer.

2. A – Abdominoperineal resection

This man has a low rectal tumour. The operative management of choice for tumours in the lower third of the rectum (within 8 cm of the anus) is abdominoperineal resection. In this procedure, the distal sigmoid colon and rectum are excised via incisions in the abdomen and perineum, with formation of an end colostomy. The anus is oversewn intraoperatively.

3. H – Sigmoid colectomy

Non-obstructing tumours of the sigmoid colon are treated with sigmoid colectomy. This operation involves removing the sigmoid colon with its blood vessels and lymph nodes, and forming an anastomosis.

4. G – Right hemicolectomy

A right hemicolectomy with primary anastomosis is the operation of choice for non-obstructed tumours of the right side of the colon. This involves removal of the distal ileum, the ascending colon and the proximal portion of the transverse colon.

5. B – Anterior resection

Tumours of the upper two-thirds of the rectum undergo anterior resection. This involves removing the rectum and usually part of the sigmoid with primary re-anastomosis between the sigmoid and lower rectum.

Tumours of the transverse colon or hepatic flexure undergo an extended right hemicolectomy. Non-obstructed tumours of the splenic flexure or descending colon are managed with left hemicolectomy.

Operative intervention is often required for inflammatory bowel disease that is unresponsive to medical treatment. In cases of terminal ileum stricturing resulting in small bowel obstruction in Crohn's disease, a stricturoplasty can be performed. In this procedure, the inflammatory strictures are incised longitudinally and then sutured transversely to widen the bowel lumen. In Crohn's disease that is mainly affecting the terminal ileum and caecum, an ileo-caecal resection is appropriate to try to preserve bowel. In patients with ulcerative colitis that is unresponsive to medical therapy, a proctocolectomy and ileo-anal pouch is the most popular operation performed, since the entire (potentially) affected bowel is being removed and a permanent ileostomy is avoided.

THEME 7: MANAGEMENT OF BREAST CANCER

1. D – Neoadjuvant chemotherapy

Surgery is the first-line treatment for breast carcinoma. Breast-conserving surgery (i.e. wide local excision) should be used where possible, although a mastectomy is required if the tumour is >4 cm in size. The woman in this scenario is keen for breast-conserving therapy, but she has a tumour that is >4 cm. In these cases, a course of neoadjuvant (i.e. presurgical) chemotherapy can be tried. This has the effect of reducing the tumour size, and may result in a tumour that is small enough to undergo wide local excision.

2. C – Modified radical mastectomy

The woman in this question has a large tumour that is >4 cm in size. This in itself is an indication for mastectomy. Mastectomy is preferable over wide local excision if the tumour is multifocal or is centrally situated. A modified radical mastectomy involves the removal of the breast, the overlying skin (including the nipple) and the axillary contents. For comparison, a radical mastectomy (unmodified) involves the removal of the pectoralis muscles *in addition* to the structures listed above.

It is worth mentioning that all patients with invasive breast carcinoma should have axillary surgery. This usually takes the form of axillary node clearance, which can be done at one of three levels. A level I clearance involves removing lymph nodes below the level of the pectoralis minor only. A level II clearance includes nodes behind the pectoralis minor, and a level III clearance incorporates the nodes above this muscle. Sentinel node biopsy is a newer technique in breast cancer surgery. The sentinel node is the first lymph node that receives lymph from the breast. It is found at operation by injecting methylene blue dye or radioactive albumin near the tumour and watching where it goes. The first lymph node it arrives at is the sentinel node, and only this is resected. If the sentinel node is found to be negative for tumour then further axillary clearance can be avoided. Sentinel node biopsy is only recommended as part of a randomized controlled trial or following an evaluated training programme.

3. E – Radiotherapy

This woman requires radiotherapy. Ipsilateral radiotherapy is given to all patients who have undergone breast-conserving surgery in order to decrease the risk of local recurrence. Radiotherapy may also be given after mastectomy for patients who have a high risk of local recurrence (i.e. large, poorly differentiated tumours or >3 positive axillary lymph nodes).

Chemotherapy can be given in some cases of breast cancer. It is considered in premenopausal women who have either node-positive disease or node-negative disease but a poorly differentiated (grade III) tumour. A typical chemotherapy regimen is the use of CMF (cyclophosphamide, methotrexate and 5-fluorouracil) given in six cycles every 3 weeks. Because the woman in this scenario has well-differentiated (grade I), node-negative disease, chemotherapy may not be considered.

4. G – Trastuzumab

Trastuzumab (Herceptin) is a monoclonal antibody that binds to the HER2 receptor (also known as ErbB-2) that may be found within some breast tumours. Activation of the HER2 receptor results in an arrest in the growth phase of mitosis, so there is reduced proliferation. Trastuzumab is only effective in tumours that express the HER2 receptor.

5. B – Aromatase inhibitor

Up to 80% of breast cancers are oestrogen or progesterone receptor positive and a further 5% of receptor negative disease will also respond to hormonal treatment. In premenopausal and postmenopausal women with oestrogen receptor-positive tumours, tamoxifen is the hormonal therapy of choice. (Tamoxifen is a selective oestrogen receptor modulator that inhibits the action of oestrogen on the tumour. Other examples include raloxifene and fluvestrant.) However, a history of venous thromboembolism is a relative contraindication to tamoxifen, and in this case an aromatase inhibitor (e.g. arimidex) is given instead. Arimidex inhibits the peripheral conversion of androgens to oestrogen by aromatase, an enzyme found in body fat. Aromatase inhibitors are only effective in postmenopausal women. This is because premenopausal women secrete large amounts of oestrogen from the ovaries and peripheral oestrogen synthesis accounts for only a small amount of total body oestrogen.

Since the woman in this scenario has a history of thromboembolism and is postmenopausal, an aromatase inhibitor would be the best option.

Other hormonal treatments of breast cancer include oophorectomy (medical or surgical). Megestrol acetate is a progesterone receptor agonist which acts by reducing the levels of circulating oestrogen.

THEME 8: TUMOUR STAGING SYSTEMS

1. G – Gleason

The Gleason score is given to prostate cancers based on their microscopic appearance. The scores range from 1 (well differentiated) to 5 (poorly differentiated). The pathologist looking at the slides identifies the two most prevalent grades (giving each a mark out of 5), and the final Gleason score is a sum of the two marks. The first number given is the predominant grade and must make up more than 51% of the sample. The final Gleason score is therefore out of 10. For example, if a prostate tumour is made up of 80% well-differentiated cells and 20% poorly differentiated cells, the final Gleason score would be 1 + 5 (or 6). The higher the score, the worse is the prognosis.

Grade 1 Prostate resembles normal tissue, small tightly packed glands
Grade 2 Well-formed glands but are less tightly packed
Grade 3 Glands are still recognizable, but evidence of invasion
Grade 4 Few recognizable glands, evidence of invasion prominent
Grade 5 No recognizable glands

Gleason score <4 has a 25% risk of progression over 10 years
Gleason score 5–7 has a 50% risk of progression over 10 years
Gleason score >7 has a 75% risk of progression over 10 years

2. C – Dukes A

The Dukes system of grading colorectal cancer was originally divided into stages A, B and C:

Dukes A Tumour is confined to the bowel wall
Dukes B Tumour invades through the bowel wall, but there is no lymph node involvement
Dukes C1 Tumour invades the bowel wall and involves local lymph nodes but proximal nodes are free from metastases
Dukes C2 Tumour invades the bowel wall and involves proximal lymph nodes

The modified Dukes system added a 'D stage' that describes the presence of distant metastases.

Five-year survival:

Dukes A: 95%
Dukes B: 80%
Dukes C1: 60%
Dukes C2: 30%
Dukes D: <5%

Cuthbert Dukes, English pathologist (1890–1977).

3. A – Ann Arbor

The Ann Arbor staging system is used for lymphomas, both Hodgkin and non-Hodgkin. The stage depends on the location of the tumour:

Stage I Lymphoma is present in one region only
Stage II Disease affects two separate groups of lymph nodes, but on one side of the diaphragm (i.e. either above or below it)
Stage III Nodes are affected both above and below the diaphragm
Stage IV Disseminated involvement of extralymphatic organs, such as the liver and bone marrow

The Ann Arbor system is named after the city of Ann Arbor in Michigan, United States, where the Committee on Hodgkin's Disease Classification met in 1971.

4. F – Dukes D

The presence of distant metastases with colorectal tumours is indicative of a Dukes D tumour.

5. B – Breslow

This woman has a malignant melanoma. The staging system used for melanomas is the Breslow depth, which is measured as the distance between the granular layer of the epidermis and the deepest point of invasion. The Breslow depth is related to prognosis.

This system was described by Alexander Breslow in 1975.

THEME 9: INVESTIGATION OF ENDOCRINE DISEASE

1. B – 24-hour urinary vanillylmandelic acid

This man presents with uncontrollable hypertension and attacks of anxiety, sweating and palpitations. Along with facial flushing and headaches, these are classic presenting features of phaeochromocytomas.

Phaeochromocytomas are tumours of the adrenal medulla (the central part of the adrenal gland). They arise from chromaffin cells and secrete large amounts of catecholamines. Breakdown products of catecholamines include vanillylmandelic acid (VMA), which is excreted in the kidney. Therefore the suspicion of phaeochromocytoma can be strengthened by finding an increased concentration of urinary VMA over a 24-hour period. An abdominal CT will help localize the tumour.

Phaeochromocytomas are associated with a 'ten-percent rule': 10% are malignant, 10% are extra-adrenal, 10% are familial and 10% are bilateral. Familial phaeochromocytomas can be associated with three main conditions: neurofibromatosis, multiple endocrine neoplasia and von Hippel-Lindau syndrome (which is characterized by phaeochromocytomas, retinal haemangioblastomas, clear cell renal carcinomas and pancreatic neuroendocrine tumours). The treatment of phaeochromocytomas is by surgical excision, but prior to this, alpha-blockers need to be given for 6 weeks to inhibit the effects of a sudden surge of catecholamines that may occur intraoperatively. A normal life expectancy is expected if treatment is successful.

2. H – Short Synacthen test

This woman presents with postural hypotension. She has vitiligo and some areas of increased skin pigmentation, making her likely to have Addison's disease. The best investigation to perform is the short Synacthen test.

Addison disease is primary autoimmune-mediated adrenocortical failure. The action of the adrenal cortex can be simplified as the secretion of three things: glucocorticoids, mineralocorticoids and adrenal androgens. These usually feed back to the anterior pituitary to reduce ACTH (adrenocorticotrophic hormone) secretion. Therefore, if the adrenal cortex fails, there are many consequences: reduced glucocorticoids (hypoglycaemia and weight loss), reduced mineralocorticoids (hyperkalaemia, hyponatraemia and hypotension), reduced adrenal androgens (decreased body hair and libido) and ACTH excess (increased pigmentation in sun-exposed areas, pressure areas, palmar creases, buccal mucosas and recent scars). The diagnosis of Addison's disease is by the short Synacthen test. In this investigation, plasma cortisol levels are measured before and half an hour after administration of a single intramuscular dose of ACTH. Normally, the ACTH will result in a rise in cortisol. If there is no rise in cortisol on the second reading, adrenal insufficiency is indicated. Management of Addison disease is by the replacement of glucocorticoids and mineralocorticoids (with hydrocortisone and fludrocortisone).

Thomas Addison, English physician (1795–1860).

3. E – Dexamethasone suppression test

This woman presents with hirsutism, striae, acne, plethora and bruising, all of which are features of Cushing syndrome. Other features include psychosis, cataracts, poor skin healing, hyperglycaemia and proximal myopathy. Because the woman has a small cell lung tumour, the cause of her Cushing syndrome could be ectopic ACTH secretion from the malignancy. The diagnosis of Cushing syndrome is by finding a raised 24-hour free urinary cortisol or with the dexamethasone suppression test (not a random cortisol, which is useless as cortisol has a natural diurnal variation). In the dexamethasone suppression test, there is a high serum cortisol level that is not suppressed by dexamethasone.

Harvey Cushing, American neurosurgeon and endocrinologist (1869–1939).

4. A – 17-Hydroxyprogesterone levels

The presentation of clitoromegaly, precocious puberty and accelerated growth in this young girl is indicative of congenital adrenal hyperplasia. Congenital adrenal hyperplasia (CAH) is an autosomal recessive deficiency in the enzyme 21-hydroxylase. This enzyme is required to synthesize mineralocorticoids and glucocorticoids (but not adrenal androgens) from the hormone precursor 17-hydroxyprogesterone. Because there is a lack of mineralocorticoids and glucocorticoids, there is no negative feedback on the anterior pituitary, resulting in increased ACTH secretion. The high ACTH then causes an increased secretion of adrenal androgens, since this does not require the deficient hormone. The androgens result in the physical features of CAH, namely ambiguous genitalia (in girls), precocious puberty (in girls), accelerated growth in childhood and virilization. The diagnosis of CAH is suggested by finding a raised concentration of the precursor 17-hydroxyprogesterone. Treatment is with hydrocortisone and fludrocortisone to replace the deficient steroids.

5. C – 24-hour urinary 5-hydroxyindole acetic acid

The features of paroxysmal flushing, diarrhoea, bronchospasm, hypo- or hypertension and abdominal pain precipitated by stress, alcohol and caffeine strongly suggest carcinoid syndrome.

Carcinoid tumours are tumours of enterochromaffin cells of the gastrointestinal tract. These enterochromoffin cells store serotonin and have a role in stimulating peristaltic movements and gut secretions. Most of these tumours arise in the appendix or small intestine (predominantly the ileum). They secrete serotonin (5-hydroxytryptamine, or 5-HT), which is carried, via the portal vein, to the liver, where it is harmlessly broken down. However, when carcinoid tumours metastasize to the liver, they can secrete 5-HT directly into the bloodstream, bypassing liver metabolism and resulting in the symptoms described above. The presence of carcinoid metastases in the liver that result in symptoms is known as carcinoid syndrome. The diagnosis of carcinoid syndrome is made by measuring 24-hour urinary 5-hydroxyindole acetic acid (5-HIAA), a breakdown product of serotonin. Management is by resection or, in widespread disease, symptomatic treatment with octreotide (a somatostatin analogue that inhibits 5-HT release). For those undergoing resection, patients are given octreotide, 5-HT antagonists and antihistamines perioperatively. During recovery, patients are carefully observed in level 2 (HDU) or level 3 (ICU) environments to facilitate careful fluid balance and blood pressure control.

Carcinoid tumours are slow-growing, so even if disseminated disease is present, patients can live for many years.

THEME 10: DIAGNOSIS OF DYSPHAGIA

1. J – Oesophageal web

This woman has anaemia with a low mean cell volume (i.e. a microcytic anaemia) as well as dysphagia. The most common cause of microcytic anaemia is iron deficiency, although other causes are thalassaemia and the anaemia of chronic disease. Chronic iron deficiency anaemia can result in hyperkeratinization of the upper oesophagus and the formation of a web that extends partially across its lumen. This is known as Plummer-Vinson syndrome (or Patterson-Brown-Kelly syndrome) and may be associated with dysphagia and odynophagia, as well as other features of iron deficiency (koilonychia and smooth tongue). Treatment of an oesophageal web is by iron supplementation with or without endoscopic dilatation of the oesophagus. Plummer-Vinson syndrome predisposes to the development of cricopharyngeal squamous cell oesophageal carcinoma.

Henry Stanley Plummer, American physician (1874–1937).

Porter Paisley Vinson, American surgeon (1890–1959).

2. K – Pharyngeal pouch

A pharyngeal pouch (or Zenker diverticulum) develops from the backward protrusion of mucosa between the inferior constrictor and cricopharyngeus muscles of the pharynx (known as Killian dehiscence). The pouch formed by the protruding mucosa initially develops posteriorly, but may later protrude to one side, usually the left, displacing the oesophagus laterally. Pharyngeal pouches are most common in older men (male:female ratio is 5:1) and present with dysphagia, regurgitation of pouch contents, halitosis, recurrent aspiration, night-time coughing and a neck swelling in the anterior triangle that gurgles on palpation. The pouch is easily visualized on barium swallow. Management is by surgical excision or stapling of the pouch. This can either be performed as an open procedure or endoscopically.

Gustav Killian, German laryngologist (1860–1921).

Friedrich von Zenker, German physician (1825–1898).

3. D – External oesophageal compression

The combination of atrial fibrillation, a flushed face and a mid-diastolic murmur suggest mitral stenosis. In context with the dysphagia, there is likely to be extrinsic oesophageal compression from an enlarged left atrium. Mitral stenosis is usually due to rheumatic fever and results in dilatation of the left atrium. Examination signs of mitral stenosis include a tapping apex beat and a low-pitched mid-diastolic murmur in the mitral area (fifth left intercostal space, mid-clavicular line).

Other causes of external oesophageal compression include an enlarged thyroid mass, aortic aneurysm, bronchial carcinoma and enlarged mediastinal lymph nodes.

4. F – Hiatus hernia

This woman has acid reflux with the appearance of an air–fluid level behind the heart. She most probably has a hiatus hernia. Risk factors included obesity, pregnancy, ascites and increasing age. There are two types of hiatus hernia: sliding (95%) and rolling (5%). In rare cases, hiatus hernias have both a sliding and a rolling element. In sliding hiatus hernias, one wall of the stomach slides up through the cardia. In rolling hiatus hernias, a portion of the stomach passes up into the thorax adjacent to the cardia. Sliding hiatus hernias are only treated if they are symptomatic. Rolling hiatus hernias require urgent surgical repair, as there is a high rate of complication (e.g. respiratory distress from lung compression or rupture of the intrathoracic stomach). The operation, a Nissen fundoplication, can usually be performed laparoscopically.

5. B – Boerhaave syndrome

This man is presenting with Boerhaave syndrome, a complete transluminal laceration (perforation) of the lower oesophagus caused by a neuromuscular failure of co-ordination to relax the upper oesophageal sphincter (cricopharyngeus muscle). It is a condition most common in middle-aged men. Oesophageal perforation most commonly occurs during endoscopy (up to 80% of cases), but other causes include spontaneous rupture following retching or trauma from a swallowed foreign body. Patients present with severe pain in the neck, chest and abdomen with dysphagia. Leakage of gastric contents into the mediastinum may cause a resultant mediastinitis that manifests as pyrexia. On examination, air may be felt in the soft tissues with a similar feel to bubble-wrap (surgical emphysema). A chest X-ray shows gas in the mediastinum, and the diagnosis is confirmed with a gastrograffin swallow. Cervical oesophageal perforations are managed conservatively (antibiotics, nil by mouth, fluids). Thoracic ruptures require immediate suture. There is a high risk of mortality, usually secondary to sepsis due to the spillage of gastric contents (pneumonitis, mediastinitis, empyema, pericarditis). A Mallory-Weiss tear is a superficial laceration in the lower oesophagus, also associated with vomiting, that results in bleeding.

Herman Boerhaave, Dutch physician (1668–1738).

THEME 11: MANAGEMENT OF URINARY RETENTION

1. J – Urethral catheterization

The presentation of acute-onset suprapubic pain, a suprapubic mass and an inability to pass urine suggests a diagnosis of acute urinary retention (ischuria). The first-line management option for acute urinary retention is the urgent passage of a urethral catheter. This patient should have his renal function checked to ensure no renal damage has occurred secondary to hydronephrosis.

2. B – Cystoscopy

This man is in acute urinary retention, most probably because a large clot has obstructed the bladder outflow. Although the initial management option would be urethral catheterization, it has failed in this case. Suprapubic catheterization is contraindicated, since the cause of the frank haematuria may be a bladder carcinoma and direct trauma to the bladder may disrupt the tumour and spread it to other parts of the tract. (Other relative contraindications to suprapubic catheterization are the presence of a bleeding tendency and previous abdominal surgery, which may result in the adhesion of small bowel to the anterior abdominal wall increasing the risk of bowel perforation.) The patient should instead undergo cystoscopic catheter insertion.

3. G – Suprapubic catheterization

This man presents with acute retention, but catheter insertion is unsuccessful. Because there are no contraindications to it, suprapubic catheter insertion should be performed. Suprapubic catheterization can be done at the bedside if the patient has a palpable bladder. In this procedure, local anaesthetic is infiltrated three finger-breadths above the pubis in the midline. As the anaesthetic is infiltrated more deeply, one should attempt to aspirate urine using the same needle. Do not proceed unless urine can be aspirated. A small incision is then made before the suprapubic catheter is inserted percutaneously and stitched to the skin.

4. I – Trial without catheter

Transurethral resection of the prostate (TURP) has been the standard management for acute urinary retention. More commonly now, however, patients are being given a trial without catheter (TWOC). In this procedure, the catheter is removed under antibiotic cover and the patient is observed with a post-micturition ultrasound and using a fluid balance chart. If the TWOC is successful then patients can be followed up as outpatients. If it is unsuccessful then the patient is considered for a TURP. TWOC is more likely to be successful if there was a predisposing factor to acute retention (e.g. constipation or a urinary tract infection) or if there was only a small residual volume (<800 mL).

5. A – Check urea and electrolytes

The presence of a palpable bladder with a long history of obstructive symptoms (hesitancy, poor stream and terminal dribbling) and overflow incontinence suggests chronic urinary retention. Chronic urinary retention is usually painless. Patients with chronic urinary retention have a residual volume >300 mL. The most common cause of chronic urinary retention is prostatic enlargement

There are two types of chronic retention: low-pressure and high-pressure. In low-pressure chronic retention, the kidney is still able to excrete urine and there is no decline in renal function. In high-pressure chronic retention, the kidney is unable to excrete urine and there is a rapid deterioration in renal function. Patients with low-pressure chronic retention should not be catheterized, as there is no rush to manage it and surgical TURP can be performed when convenient. Catheterization will only risk introducing infection to a sterile system. Patients with high-pressure chronic retention will need urgent decompression of their renal tract to prevent further kidney damage, so urgent catheterization is indicated. The way to differentiate between low- and high-pressure systems is to measure the urea and electrolytes, which will only be deranged in high-pressure chronic retention.

THEME 12: DIAGNOSIS OF PAEDIATRIC SURGICAL CONDITIONS

1. B – Duodenal atresia

Duodenal atresia is the congenital absence or closure of a portion of the duodenum. Around one-third of babies with duodenal atresia have trisomy 21 (Down syndrome). Affected babies present at birth with bile-stained vomiting and abdominal distension. Diagnosis is confirmed by the presence of a double-bubble sign on the abdominal X-ray. This represents the presence of air in the stomach and proximal duodenum only, and not in the distal intestines. Treatment is by duodenoduodenostomy.

2. E – Hirschprung disease

Hirschprung disease is a congenital absence of ganglion cells (aganglionosis) from both the myenteric (Auerbach) plexus and submucosal (Meissner) plexus of the large bowel, resulting in a narrowed, contracted segment. The abnormally innervated bowel extends proximally from the rectum for a variable distance. Hirschprung disease often presents in neonates with abdominal distension and bile-stained vomiting. Rectal examination shows a narrowed segment, and removal of the examining finger is often followed by a gush of stools and flatus. Occasionally, Hirschprung disease can present in childhood with chronic constipation and abdominal distension without soiling. Diagnosis is by rectal biopsy, which demonstrates the absence of ganglion cells in the affected mucosa. Management is by excision of the abnormal bowel (rectosigmoidectomy), with re-anastomosis to the anus (coloanal anastomisis). A defunctioning stoma may also be sited. Like duodenal atresia, Hirschprung disease is also associated with Down syndrome.

Harald Hirschprung, Danish paediatrician (1830–1916).

Leopold Auerbach, German neuropathologist (1828–1897).

Georg Meissner, German anatomist (1829–1905).

3. D – Gastroschisis

Gastroschisis is a defect in the anterior abdominal wall adjacent to the umbilicus. Abdominal contents, such as the liver and intestines, can herniate through this defect, but there is no sac covering the contents. Management of gastroschisis is by immediately covering the exposed viscera with clingfilm, followed by operative repair. Gastroschisis is rarely associated with other congenital malformations.

Gastroschisis, from Greek *gastro* = belly + *schisis* = cleft; 'split belly'.

Exomphalos is the herniation of abdominal contents through the umbilicus. The herniated viscera are surrounded by a sac (the amnion); this structure is known as an omphalocele. Surgical closure of the defect is required. Fifty percent of cases of exomphalos are associated with other congenital malformations, such as trisomies and cardiac defects.

4. A – Appendicitis

Acute appendicitis is the most common surgical emergency in childhood. Inflammation of the appendix occurs secondary to obstruction of the appendiceal opening into the caecum. Obstruction can be by a faecolith, adhesions or lymphoid hyperplasia. Abdominal pain is initially central (the appendix is a midgut structure, so pain is referred to the umbilicus) but later shifts to the right iliac fossa due to localized peritonitis. Patients also have anorexia, nausea and vomiting and a low-grade fever. Classically, there is pain over McBurney's point, which is found one-third of the way between the anterior superior iliac spine and the umbilicus. Rovsing sign, where palpation over the left iliac fossa causes right iliac fossa pain, may also be positive. If the inflamed appendix is adjacent to the bladder or rectum, dysuria or diarrhoea can feature. Leucocytes may also be seen on urine analysis due to the ureter's close proximity. Although the diagnosis of appendicitis is a clinical one, the Alvarado or Mantrel score may be used to quantify how likely the diagnosis is. This scoring system is based on history: 1 point each for migratory pain, anorexia (or ketones in urine), nausea or vomiting, examination (right iliac fossa tenderness, rebound tenderness, fever) and laboratory findings (leukocytosis, neutrophilia). A maximum score of 10 can be achieved, with 2 points being awarded to leukocytosis and right iliac fossa tenderness.

Management is by appendicectomy.

Faecolithm, from Latin *faeco* = excrement + Greek *lith* = stone; 'piece of poo'.

Charles McBurney, American surgeon (1845–1913).

Niels Thorkild Rovsing, Danish surgeon (1862–1927).

5. G – Meckel diverticulum

Meckel diverticulum is a congenital diverticulum that contains gastric-type mucosa. It is an example of a true diverticulum. A true diverticulum incorporates all the layers of the wall from which it arises. False diverticula are made up of only the inner layer of the normal bowel wall, an example being colonic diverticula. There is a rule of twos regarding Meckel diverticulum: it is found 2 feet proximal to the ileo-caecal junction, it is 2 inches in length and it occurs in 2% of the population. Most Meckel diverticula are incidental findings, but the most common presentation is painless rectal bleeding. Some may present with acute inflammation, similar to acute appendicitis. Because Meckel diverticula contain gastric mucosa, they are susceptible to peptic ulceration. Diagnosis is confirmed by a technetium-99m scan. The technetium radiolabel is taken up only by gastric-type mucosa, so the scan will highlight the stomach as well as a diverticulum in the right iliac fossa. Treatment is by resection if required.

Diverticulum, from Latin *diverticulum* = byroad.

Johann Friedrich Meckel, German anatomist (1781–1833).

THEME 13: DIAGNOSIS OF FOOT DISORDERS

1. C – Gout

Gout occurs secondary to deposition of uric acid crystals in the joint. It is most common in older, obese male drinkers with hypertension, ischaemic heart disease and diabetes. Other risk factors include cytotoxic drugs, diuretic use and Lesch-Nyhan syndrome (gout + mental retardation + self-mutilating behaviour). Acute gout usually presents with sudden pain, swelling and redness in the first metatarsophalangeal joint, although 25% of cases occur in the knee. Diagnosis is by joint aspiration, which shows negatively birefringent needle-shaped crystals. Acute gout is treated with NSAIDs (e.g. indometacin or diclofenac). Prophylaxis is with allopurinol, axanthine oxidase inhibitor that slows the production of uric acid. This is offered to patients who have recurrent or chronic gout, who are receiving cytotoxic therapy, or who have Lesch-Nyhan syndrome.

Pseudogout is caused by the deposition of calcium pyrophosphate in the joint and results in features similar to gout. It occurs most commonly in older women and usually affects the knee or wrist. Joint aspiration in pseudogout shows weakly positively birefringent brick-shaped crystals. Acute pseudogout is treated with NSAIDs. No prophylactic therapy is available.

The important differential diagnosis in a hot, erythematous joint is septic arthritis. If in doubt, blood tests should be taken for inflammatory markers, X-rays taken and the joint aspirated. This fluid should be sent for urgent Gram staining to look for the presence of bacteria.

2. I – Morton metatarsalgia

Morton metatarsalgia describes a neuroma of the interdigital nerve between the third and fourth toes (although it can occur between other toes). Patients describe a sharp pain in the web space at this area that radiates to the toes. Diagnosis is confirmed by USS or MRI. Surgical excision of the neuroma is curative.

Thomas Morton, American surgeon (1835–1903).

3. K – Sever disease

Sever disease is an apophysitis at the calcaneus (similar to Osgood-Schlatter disease of the tibial tuberosity). It is the most common cause of heel pain in children between 8 and 14 years and is caused by inflammation of the growth plate. Features include heel pain, which is worse after exercise, and limping. The mainstay of treatment is rest, and most cases resolve spontaneously within a few weeks.

Freiberg disease is an osteochondritis of the second or third metatarsals. Osteochondritis is characterized by patchy avascular necrosis and reactive sclerosis of an area of bone, which can result in collapse and fragmentation. Eventually there is regrowth of the bone. X-ray of the affected bone shows it to be dense and flat. Patients present with severe localized pain in the affected area. Other examples of osteochondritis are Kienbock disease (lunate), Scheurmann disease (spine) and Perthes disease (hip).

4. H – March fracture

A march fracture is an undisplaced hairline fracture that usually affects the second or third metatarsal near its neck. It is caused by a history of repeated stress – hence the name. Features include severe pain in the forefoot on walking and callus formation at the site of the fracture. Treatment is with analgesia, and the pain resolves after a few weeks when fracture union occurs.

5. E – Hallux valgus

Hallux valgus is a lateral deviation of the great toe that is relatively common in women past middle age. It is caused by the toe being persistently forced laterally by wearing narrow shoes. Over several years, bunions (a thick-walled bursa) and osteoarthritis can develop over the metatarsal head. Surgical intervention is required in severe cases.

Hallus valgus, from Latin *hallex* = great toe.

Bunion, from Latin *bunio* = turnip.

Hallux rigidus is osteoarthritis of the metatarsophalangeal (MTP) joint of the great toe. A hammer toe is a fixed flexion deformity of an interphalangeal joint. The proximal interphalangeal (PIP) joint is in fixed flexion and the distal interphalangeal (DIP) joint rests in compensatory hyperextension. A callosity usually forms on the dorsal aspect of the affected toes due to pressure from shoes. Hammer toe is most common in the second digit and is usually associated with hallux valgus. A mallet toe is a flexion deformity of the DIP joint, with normal MTP and PIP joints. Claw toes involve MTP extension, PIP flexion and DIP flexion. Claw toes result from weakness of the intrinsic muscles of the foot, which normally extend the PIP and DIP joints. Causes of clawing include rheumatoid arthritis, poor footwear and underlying neurological disease (e.g. poliomyelitis or Friedreich ataxia).

THEME 14: DIAGNOSIS OF ABDOMINAL PAIN

1. A – Acute appendicitis

This patient is presenting with classic features of acute appendicitis. If at laparoscopy the appendix appears macroscopically normal, an alternative diagnosis should be sought. These include a ruptured ovarian cyst, Crohn's disease, Meckel diverticulitis and pelvic inflammatory disease.

2. I – Osler-Weber-Rendu syndrome

Osler-Weber-Rendu syndrome (also known as hereditary haemorrhagic telangiectasia) is an autosomal dominant condition characterized by multiple telangiectasias around the mouth and gastrointestinal tract, along with recurrent painless bleeding (epistaxis or GI bleeding is the most common presentation but lesions can occur at other sites). The majority of patients present by the age of 40. It is a rare condition with a prevalence of 10 per 100,000 people. Diagnosis requires three of the following criteria: recurrent spontaneous epistaxis; multiple visible telangiectasias; the presence of internal telangiectasias and arteriovenous malformations; and having an affected first-degree relative. Because of recurrent bleeding, many patients have anaemia that requires multiple blood transfusions.

This patient presented with abdominal pain. Although bleeding in Osler-Weber-Rendu syndrome tends to be painless, abdominal pain can occur if there is thrombosis of an alimentary arteriovenous malformation.

Sir William Osler, Canadian physician (1849–1919).
Frederick Parkes Weber, English physician (1863–1962).
Henri Jules Rendu, French physician (1844–1902).

3. H – Mesenteric angina

Mesenteric angina is a postprandial severe abdominal pain that occurs due to atherosclerosis of the blood supply to the bowel, similar to what angina is to the heart. The pain occurs after eating because the demands of the bowel are increased. Pain begins 10 minutes after eating and can last around half an hour. Affected patients tend to avoid food, and stigmata of weight loss may be evident on examination. During an episode, the abdomen is surprisingly soft. Risk factors for mesenteric angina are similar to those for any atherosclerotic condition: smoking, obesity, diabetes, hypertension, hypercholesterolaemia, etc. The diagnosis can be confirmed by mesenteric angiography, which shows narrowing of the affected mesenteric artery. Treatment is by 'best medical therapy', including statins and aspirin, and angioplasty with stent insertion will improve symptoms.

4. C – Acute radiation enterocolitis

The treatment of many tumours involves radiotherapy. Acute radiation enterocolitis describes the sloughing of the dead epithelial lining of the bowel wall. Symptoms can occur within hours of starting radiotherapy, but most often begin 3 weeks into treatment. Clinical features include anorexia, nausea, vomiting, abdominal cramps, watery diarrhoea and rectal bleeding. This acute radiation injury is self-limiting and management is symptomatic. Chronic radiation enterocolitis develops months or years after therapy. It is caused by transmural bowel damage and resultant destruction of end arteries. Features include small bowel structuring and obstruction, malabsorption, and fistula development. It is a progressive disease that is difficult to treat.

5. F – Ectopic pregnancy

Ectopic pregnancy affects 1% of pregnancies and results when a fertilized ovum implants outside the uterus. Most ectopic pregnancies are found in the Fallopian tubes. Risk factors include pelvic inflammatory disease, previous ectopy, tube ligation and the presence of an intrauterine contraceptive device. An ectopic pregnancy presents initially as a missed period. When the ectopic ruptures, there is severe, crampy lower abdominal pain with guarding and rebound tenderness. Bleeding from the ruptured ectopic can result in shock. Vaginal examination is contraindicated in suspect ectopic pregnancies, as it may provoke haemorrhage. A urinary β-hCG test will confirm pregnancy and help differentiate a ruptured ectopic pregnancy from other causes of acute abdomen. If haemorrhage has not already occurred, management is with methotrexate. The patient in this scenario has signs of haemorrhagic shock, so urgent laparoscopy or laparotomy with ectopic removal is required.

Any female of child-bearing age presenting with abdominal pain should have her urine tested for β-hCG. Assume all women of this age to be pregnant until proven otherwise.

THEME 15: MANAGEMENT OF HEAD INJURY

1. C – Home with written advice

It should be noted that a brief loss of consciousness (<5 minutes) and fully resolved post-traumatic amnesia are not indications for admission following head injury.

Admission criteria include:

- Loss of consciousness lasting >5 minutes
- Confusion or decreased GCS

- Skull fracture
- Neurological signs or symptoms
- Intoxication (e.g. with alcohol or drugs)
- Worsening headache, nausea or vomiting
- No responsible adult at home
- Other medical comorbidities

It is appropriate to send this patient home with verbal and written advice under the responsibility of another adult. He should be warned of possible complications and told what to do if his condition deteriorates.

2. E – Refer to neurosurgery

A depressed skull fracture is an indication for neurosurgical opinion. Other criteria include a skull fracture in the presence of neurological signs, confusion persisting for >12 hours and deterioration of GCS.

3. A – Admit for neurological observation

The presence of a skull fracture and intoxication are criteria for admission for neurological observation following head injury (see above list).

4. D – Intubation and ventilation

This woman has a GCS of 3 and thus will be unable to protect her airway. Intubation and ventilation is essential in this case.

5. B – CT head scan

The presence of cerebrospinal fluid (CSF) leaking from the nose indicates a basal skull fracture. Basal skull fractures are rare and involve a linear fracture at the base of the skull. CSF otorrhoea (from the ear) and CSF rhinorrhoea (from the nose) are pathognomonic of such fractures. Other features to look out for are Battle sign (bruising of the mastoid process of the temporal bone), raccoon eyes (periorbital bruising) and haemotympanum (the presence of blood behind the tympanic membrane). A suspected basal skull fracture requires a CT head scan.

The following is a list of indications for urgent neuroimaging:

GCS <13 on initial assessment in the emergency department

GCS <15 two hours after the injury on assessment in the emergency department

Suspected open or depressed skull fracture

Any sign of basal skull fracture, e.g.

- Haemotympanum (blood behind the tympanic membrane)
- 'Panda eyes' (bilateral periorbital ecchymosis caused by blood from ruptured venous sinuses tracking into the cranial sinuses, aka 'raccoon eyes')
- Bilateral subconjunctival haemorrhage
- CSF leakage from ears (CSF otorrhoea) or nose (CSF rhinorrhoea)
- Battle's sign (perimastoid ecchymosis from extravasation of blood along the path of the posterior auricular artery)

Post-traumatic seizure
Focal neurological deficit
>1 episode of vomiting
Amnesia for events more than 30 minutes before the injury

William Henry Battle, English surgeon (1855–1936).

THEME 16: UROLOGICAL CONDITIONS

1. G – Prostate carcinoma

The features of hesitancy and terminal dribbling with a percussable (enlarged) bladder suggest bladder outflow obstruction, which could be benign prostatic hyperplasia or prostate carcinoma. This man also suffered a back injury on minimal trauma, implying a pathological fracture from metastatic invasion of the bone, which could only be due to underlying prostate carcinoma. Metastases to bone tend to occur at haematopoetic sites (spine, pelvis, ribs, skull and proximal long bones). They are either osteosclerotic (prostate or breast) or osteolytic (lung, renal, colon, melanoma).

2. A – Acute cystitis

Acute cystitis is inflammation of the bladder, which is most common in sexually active women. Females are more prone to developing cystitis due to their shorter urethra. Other risk factors for developing cystitis include tumours, instrumentation of the bladder and the presence of residual urine in the bladder after voiding (e.g. with bladder outflow obstruction). Most cases are caused by *Escherichia coli* from the gastrointestinal tract. Other causes include *Proteus* and *Pseudomonas.* Proteus infections will cause alkaline urine due to the organism's ability to split urea into NH_3 and CO_2. Patients present with dysuria, frequency and nocturia, and may have haematuria or cloudy, offensive urine. A urine dipstick may show blood, protein, leukocytes and nitrites. A mid-stream urine (MSU) sample can be sent to culture bacteria and determine appropriate antibiotic sensitivities. The presence of leukocytes in the urine with $>10^5$ organisms/mL on MSU and characteristic clinical features confirms the diagnosis. A typical initial management regimen for acute cystitis is trimethoprim 200 mg twice daily for 3 days.

Pyelonephritis occurs when pathogens ascend the ureters from the bladder. Patients present with symptoms of cystitis with the addition of fever, nausea/vomiting and costal angle tenderness. Although nitrofurantoin is commonly used in the treatment of urinary tract infections, it is contraindicated in pyelonephritis because it does not achieve adequate renal tissue levels.

3. C – Benign prostatic hyperplasia

Benign enlargement of the prostate is common after the age of 45 under the influence of hormones. In fact, 70% of men have benign hyperplasia

by the age of 70. Prostatic hyperplasia results in bladder outflow obstruction that presents with hesitancy, poor stream and terminal dribbling. There may also be haematuria at the end of the stream as the bladder contracts around the enlarged prostate. Eventually, the bladder becomes completely obstructed and urinary retention can result. On examination, an enlarged bladder may be palpable and dull to percussion. A per rectum exam will exhibit a smooth, enlarged prostate.

4. D – Bladder neck stenosis

Worsening lower urinary tract symptoms following a transurethral resection of the prostate suggests a stricture at the bladder neck, a recognized complication of the operation.

5. E – Nephroblastoma

A nephroblastoma (or Wilms tumour) is an anaplastic malignant tumour arising from embryonic mesodermal tissues, occurring under the age of 5 years. It is associated with a deletion on the short arm of chromosome 11 and may be linked with other congenital anomalies (e.g. macroglossia and aniridia). Spread occurs early to regional nodes and to the lung and liver. Patients present with a loin mass, weight loss, anorexia and fever. Haematuria is a rarer sign, as renal pelvis involvement is late. Treatment is by resection (if possible) and radiotherapy, with an 80% survival rate at 5 years. Nephroblastomas are pale grey with areas of haemorrhage on cross-section.

Max Wilms, German surgeon (1867–1918).

THEME 17: MANAGEMENT OF ABDOMINAL AORTIC ANEURYSMS

The normal size of the abdominal aorta is 2 cm. A dilatation of the abdominal aorta to >3 cm is defined as an abdominal aortic aneurysm (AAA). AAAs are more common in men, affecting 5% of those aged over 65. Other risk factors are smoking, hypertension, hypercholesterolaemia and family history. The majority of AAAs (95%) are below the renal arteries (infrarenal) and 30% extend to involve the iliac arteries below.

AAAs are relatively common, with a prevalence of 1.4% in the United States. Patients can present with a variety of symptoms ranging from unimpressive groin, flank, back or abdominal pain to catastrophic cardiovascular collapse. While symptoms of pain can be insidious in onset, many AAAs are asymptomatic and the associated mortality with rupture is high.

1. B – Emergency surgery

This man presents with features of shock and epigastric pain radiating to the back. This is a typical presentation of a ruptured AAA. This patient should be taken to theatre as an emergency (after gaining intravenous access and taking basic bloods, including a crossmatch). A CT or ultrasound scan should only be performed if the diagnosis is in doubt, for example if a known drinker presents with epigastric pain radiating to the back, in which case pancreatitis would be in the differential. Patients who are haemodynamically unstable should not be taken to CT. Most people with ruptured AAAs die before reaching hospital. Fifty percent of those who make it die within the next 30 days.

2. G – Ultrasound in 1 year

AAAs that are asymptomatic and <4 cm in size should have annual ultrasound surveillance.

3. F – Ultrasound in 6 months

AAAs that are asymptomatic and between 4 and 5.5 cm in size should undergo 6-monthly ultrasound surveillance.

4. E – Urgent elective repair

A rapid increase in size of >1 cm in an AAA is an indication for urgent elective repair. The other indication for urgent elective repair is the development of symptoms associated with the AAA. Symptomatic aneurysms are usually rapidly expanding or leaking.

5. D – Elective open repair

Indications for elective repair of an AAA are an increase in size to >5.5 cm or an aneurysm that expands >1 cm in one year. The mortality rate for elective repair is 5%, compared with a risk of rupture of 5% per year. Elective repair can be performed as an open procedure or an endoluminal procedure.

Endoluminal repair involves passing a vascular graft into the aorta via the femoral artery. This technique is only suitable when the AAA begins >3 cm below the renal arteries. If this is not the case, open repair is required. The elective mortality rate for open AAA repair is 5%.

Index

D

E

F

G

H

Index

R

S

T

U

V

W

Z